MEDICINE,
MARATHONS
&MIRACLES

MEDICINE, MARATHONS & MIRACLES

Turning a Diagnosis of Cancer into Personal Victory

Kathy & Roger Cawthon

With an introduction by Bernie S. Siegel, M.D.
New York Times Bestselling Author of
Love, Medicine and Miracles and *Peace, Love and Healing*

Published by
Ruby ❖ Press

MEDICINE, MARATHONS & MIRACLES
Turning a Diagnosis of Cancer into Personal Victory

Copyright © 2005 Kathy and Roger Cawthon

Published by
Ruby ❖ Press
Hampton, Virginia

Printed in the United States of America

ISBN # 0-9770773-0-6

You gain strength, courage and confidence every time
you really stop to look fear in the face...You *must* do
the thing you think you cannot do.

– Eleanor Roosevelt

* * * * *

The race belongs not only to the swift and the strong,
but also to those who keep running.

– Author Unknown

Authors' Note

For the sake of clarity and for ease of reading, this book is written in the first person from Kathy's viewpoint, even though this story is *our* story.

The names of doctors and some other individuals have been changed to protect their privacy.

Dedication

This book is dedicated with great love and gratitude to our families who were beside us every step of the way throughout our cancer experience, especially Fred and Clara Mayfield, Jim and Gwen Cawthon, Mary Priddy, Charlsie Brown, Ryan Corbett and Reid Corbett;

To John Q.A. Mattern, Eric M. Bashkoff and Bishop P. Read for saving our lives. There are no words that can express the depth of our gratitude to you, so we humbly offer up this dedication as our small "thank you" for the immeasurable gift of a second chance at life;

To "myfriendkathy" who is fighting (and winning!) the good fight as this book goes to print. You are without question the strongest, most courageous person I have ever known, and the sister I never had but always wished for. Let me know when you're ready to run your marathon. I'll be right there beside you;

And to every cancer survivor everywhere. Always know that you are not alone in your battle. You are a warrior in an army of millions. Fight on.

The Big "C"

by Kathy Cawthon, Survivor

*"The big 'C'" I heard someone call it.
Another just whispered the word.
That we don't even dare to say "cancer" out loud
Gives it power it doesn't deserve.*

*So I'm giving that letter new meaning
And refusing to give in to fear
By reclaiming the power for you and for me
And by saying these words loud and clear:*

*Let the "C" be for "Cure" and "Compassion."
Let it stand for the "Candles" we light,
And a "Chorus" of voices shouting, "You 'Can'!"
To all who will take up this fight.*

*Let the "C" be for "Cash Contribution"
("Credit" or "Check" will work, too).
Let it stand for "Commitment" and "Checkups"
        and "Cheer,"
And the "Children" "Counting" on you.*

*Let it mean that we know our "Creator"
Is beside us each step of the way,
And remind us to "Call" on His strength and
        His love
And to "Celebrate" every new day.*

*To everyone facing this "Challenge,"
I say it's a fight we can win.
Tell all who will listen that, starting today,
The "C" is for "Courage," my friend.*

Table of Contents

Introduction

I ran my first marathon because the father of a boy with leukemia asked me to help him raise funds to find a cure. Today, millions of dollars have been raised by people running marathons in the race to cure leukemia.

The day before I wrote this, our son and daughter-in-law ran in the New York Marathon. At the starting line, our son was standing next to two brothers. Their conversation revealed that one of the brothers had just finished his battle with cancer and was now challenging himself by running the marathon. Our son was greatly inspired by the two men.

Many marathoners will tell you the most important goal they have is to finish. The time it takes is not the issue. All finishers are winners, and everyone who finishes receives a medal. At every marathon, spectators can be heard cheering the runners on by calling out, "You're all winners!" As one injured athlete said as he struggled to complete the marathon, "I didn't come to quit. I came to finish."

And so it is with life. How many years one lives is not the issue; what you accomplish in those years is. Each person's personal marathon is about confronting the challenge of life and creating miracles through love because the only thing of permanence *is* love. Even marathon record times fall, but love stands for all eternity.

I am often disturbed when I read or hear that someone has "lost his battle with cancer." To me dying is not failing or losing, just as not being first in the marathon doesn't make you a loser. Death is not a failure but a chance to leave a tired body just as one rests after the marathon.

As Ruth Gordon said in the movie *Harold and Maude*, "Give me an L! Give me an I! Give me a V! Give me an E! Live! Otherwise, you've got nothing to talk about in the locker room."

So it is with cancer. The will to live and challenge their disease turns cancer patients into winners who can teach us all how to survive. We all need coaches to guide us, and those who take on the marathon of cancer become some of our best guides and teachers. They show us how to finish what we started and how to burn up and not out. They live their lives to the fullest, and there is no candle left when they are done.

This book will bring you to tears and joy as it did me. Those feelings let me know that it is real and honest and contains many truths about life. It is all about achieving personal victories, victories that have nothing to do with "winning" or "losing". The Cawthons' story has the power to inspire readers to set and achieve goals that will amaze themselves and everyone around them.

There is no guilt, shame or blame in the authors' depiction of life. They know the world is imperfect so that our acts are meaningful and help creation to occur. They know a perfect world is a magic trick without meaning, just as everyone finishing the marathon in two hours would be. They know how to find the blessing in the curse and that the blessings are all the things that help us to complete ourselves. They know that sometimes the blessings don't feel very good in the same way that a runner may not feel very good at about the twentieth mile of a marathon.

And they know that – under great pressure – a lump of coal can be transformed into a diamond.

What we all need to realize is that life is about beginnings. When you experience loss or disaster, you must begin again if you are to survive. It takes a lot of courage to accept a new challenge, and it takes inspiration – not just information – to accomplish that. If you are not inspired, it doesn't matter how much you know because you will not use it to change your life. Just as the marathon runner needs to train and to breathe to supply his or her body with oxygen, we need to inspire ourselves to awaken and vitalize our minds, our spirits and our bodies and give them the will to live.

Find the rhythm in your life just as a runner finds his pace. By finding rhythm, you will free your mind and body to perform at the peak of their abilities. The rhythm is different for each of us.

So create your own orchestra and lead it. Play your own song, and don't waste time trying to avoid the inevitable. Do try to achieve the unusual – a meaningful life – and teach others about survival behavior as you cross the finish line.

Choose your own "marathon" and train every day to become the person you want to be. Every athlete and actor knows that it takes rehearsing and practicing to become a star performer. The key is to not criticize your performance, but rather to keep practicing and moving forward, knowing that you *will* cross the finish line some day where your medal will be waiting for you because you are a winner.

Bernie S. Siegel, M.D.

Foreword

John Lennon once said, "Life is what happens to you while you're busy making other plans."

Truer words were never spoken.

It certainly was true in his life. A gifted and immensely popular musician, poet and artist, Lennon had found his soul mate in artist Yoko Ono, and together they had a healthy, beautiful son. Life was good, and the future looked brighter than ever. Book and movie deals, new recording contracts, gallery exhibits – those were their plans.

Until life happened.

On a cold, drizzly evening in New York City, December 8, 1980, John Lennon was shot and killed outside his Central Park apartment by a crazed fan.

We are all familiar with other names of well-known people who seemed to have their whole lives ahead of them, whose futures held great promise but were cut tragically short. Princess Diana and John F. Kennedy, Jr. are two of the most obvious examples.

The actor Christopher Reeve was surely making other plans when he was thrown from his horse during a riding exhibition in 1995. Life happened in one terrible moment, and he went from being the man everyone knew as the movie hero Superman to a quadriplegic dependent on others for every breath he took. He died from the combined and long-term effects of his injuries nine years later.

Nearly three thousand Americans were making other plans when they went to work or boarded airplanes on September 11, 2001. Their lives ended that day, and the lives of countless thousands of others, their families and friends – who also were making other plans – were forever changed by the nightmare now known simply as "9/11."

All of these people and the tragedies that befell them made headlines around the world either because of the celebrity status of those involved or the sheer enormity of the event.

But life happens to ordinary individuals making other plans every single day, quietly and with little or no warning, in doctors' offices and clinics and hospitals around the world. Someone says the word "cancer" and, in an instant, someone else's life changes forever.

A diagnosis of cancer impacts everyone connected to the patient: family members and friends, co-workers and acquaintances, doctors and nurses. Even the pathologist – who has never met the patient and who, in his sterile lab environment, peers through the lens of his microscope and makes the horrible discovery – probably experiences a quickening heartbeat and dread of the report he must make.

But the impact it makes on the patient himself (if he is of sufficient years to understand the diagnosis) cannot be measured in heartbeats or breaths or tears. In the instant he hears the word "cancer," the plans he was making seem to vanish in the air like bubbles from a child's plastic wand.

No matter how many loved ones surround and support him, no matter how many assurances he receives from medical professionals that there are new treatments to try and miracles on the horizon, no matter how many stories he hears or reads of spontaneous remissions and answered prayers, the patient who has received a diagnosis of cancer feels suspended in time and space, completely alone, set adrift on a sea of uncertainty and fear. The realization that his life will never, ever be the same again is a cruel blow to even the strongest spirit. And the knowledge that this disease could mean the end of his life is enough to bring the most stoic individual to his knees.

There are, of course, those rare individuals who, by some quirk of personality or by the power of tremendous religious faith, are able to bear up rather well when they receive a diagnosis of cancer. Others may *seem* to be bearing up well when they have actually retreated into denial.

We did not have either that quirk of personality or tremendous religious faith, and we did not and could not deny what was happening to us.

My husband and I were diagnosed with cancer within six weeks of one another.

Life happened while we were making other plans.

We had two teenage sons from my first marriage, busy careers and dreams for the future, both for the boys and for ourselves. Roger, a successful contractor and former television sportscaster, longed to combine his talents by creating and leading business seminars and by speaking professionally at sales conferences and conventions. I had worked for years as a freelance journalist and photographer, and I dreamed of the day when I would have time to write the novels that constantly played out in my head and create works of photographic art rather than the day-to-day story-related assignments that consumed most of my time. We dreamed of one day moving to a cottage at the shore where I could write and create and where Roger's speaking career could be headquartered.

We dreamed of the boys finding their way in the world, discovering their life partners, of their weddings and babies, and of all of us living and loving happily ever after.

Then someone said the word "cancer."

And it seemed the world stopped spinning.

How did it happen? How had our lives come to this? Why both of us at the same time?

We had always been healthy, and we just assumed we would always *be* healthy.

The simple truth was that we had taken our good health for granted and abused our bodies in many ways. With the dual diagnoses of cancer came the horrible realization that now it was too late. We couldn't go back and undo the things we had done or that had happened to us. We could only deal with the reality of what was.

Dealing with that reality and coming to terms with the impact of cancer on our lives would consume many months and years to come.

While we had wonderful support from the medical community and from family and friends, most of what we learned was through trial and error, countless missteps, and more frustration, anger and tears than we care to remember. Some of the anguish was normal and necessary, *but much of it was not.*

Today we have a theory that life on earth is a cosmic schoolroom and that, to become our very best selves and to give our very best to the world, we have to learn some hard lessons. And, in spite of what some people might believe, those lessons are *not* punishment for past transgressions or failure to pay attention to the Teacher.

In addition, we have a choice as to how we handle the lessons. We can let them destroy us, or we can learn to see them as extra help, extra gifts, extra blessings that can make us healthier, stronger and better in every way *if* we take advantage of what they have to teach us.

During our illnesses and recoveries, a lot of people said to us, "Remember that God won't give you more than you can handle."

We cringed when people said that because, even though we weren't regular churchgoers or "religious" in the sense that many have of that word, we believe in God and we believe that He is a gentle, loving Father. Gentle, loving fathers don't hurt and kill their children. We never believed – not for a single minute – that God gave us cancer any more than we believe that God directed a madman to kill John Lennon, pushed Christopher Reeve from his horse or instructed terrorists to fly airplanes into buildings.

What we came to believe is that God is the warm and loving Teacher in that great cosmic classroom. He is there to comfort and guide us through the lessons and to help us with the hard parts, but the lessons themselves are determined by many things: biology, accidents, our own actions and the evil that others do.

We have developed these beliefs during the ten years that have passed since our cancer diagnoses.

Our intent in writing this book is twofold: to inspire and motivate cancer patients to move from being "victims" to being "victors"; and to illustrate that *miracles really do happen* and that sometimes we experience them in the middle of the most unlikely circumstances.

This book is the story of our journey from sickness to health, from a life of stress to one of peace, from bitterness to joy, and from terror to faith.

The journey is different for everyone, but our greatest hope is that we can make yours a more comfortable and less frightening one by sharing the lessons we've learned along the way.

We hope we can help you see that a diagnosis of cancer is not just a confrontation with your mortality, but oh, so much more. It is the *opportunity* to make peace with your mortality and then to use that peace to live every moment of the rest of your life with unlimited joy and passion.

MEDICINE...

Chapter 1

Life Before Cancer

Roger and I had been married for thirteen years when cancer entered our lives. Our marriage had been a strong one from the beginning, but our family life had been chaotic and had contained its share of tragedy. Sometimes family members commented that it felt like we were living in a soap opera.

Several close relatives had battled addiction problems, depression and other emotional difficulties and had been in and out of treatment facilities. We had lain awake countless nights worrying about people we loved, simultaneously waiting for the phone to ring and fearing that it would. We were summoned to the hospital on several occasions along with other family members to wait to learn whether a loved one would live or die from an overdose or suicide attempt.

My first marriage had been a disastrous one, and both of my sons suffered from the aftereffects of that tumultuous time as evidenced by behavioral problems both at home and school. The boys' biological father and I remained embroiled in bitter custody and support issues that seemed to have no end.

In 1990, my younger brother Tom died of AIDS. We had learned of his illness only a year before his death, and that year took a heavy emotional toll on the entire family. Back then, a diagnosis of AIDS meant certain death in almost every case. I began grieving as soon as we knew he was sick, but both my mother and father believed a miracle cure would be found in time.

In the last months of his life, Tom came home to be with our family. He moved between my parents' home and ours, but the time came when none of us could care for him any longer. We simply did not have the equipment, supplies, expertise or experience to make him comfortable. To our disappointment, we learned the local hospitals and their affiliated hospices did not offer much in the way of patient or family services in cases of AIDS.

Finally, we heard about a former priest who had purchased a private home and opened it as a hospice for AIDS patients. We contacted him, and Tom was invited to "Jack's House." He spent his last three weeks there, surrounded by loving family and friends and supported by caring professionals. A compassionate physician made regular rounds and wrote prescriptions. Nurses and student nurses took turns stopping by to help bathe the patients and provide other comforting measures. Specially trained hospice workers from another city volunteered their time at "Jack's House," too, and helped patients and their loved ones prepare for the inevitable.

I was with my brother when he died on March 15, 1990. It was a beautiful spring morning, and gentle breezes came through the two open windows in his room. A nurse told me to hold him and talk to him softly. I did, and his passing was, I believe, peaceful for him. I know it was a sacred moment for me. In the few minutes after he died, I felt his presence around me, literally touching and comforting me, letting me know that he had left us to go somewhere where he would be well and whole and where we would all be together again some day.

Still, his death was a blow to the family. Adding to our tremendous sense of loss was the lack of open and honest communication about AIDS in our community. We felt isolated and lonely in our grief.

I had resigned from my teaching position to spend more time with my brother and with my sons, hoping to help the children better cope with the chaos created by their father, their uncle's illness and other family issues. I began doing some freelance writing and photography for several local newspapers and magazines, but the pay fell far short of my previous salary. We began to struggle financially as we had never done before, but agreed it was more important for me to be there for the children and my brother than to return to working full-time.

Clearly, our family was experiencing its share of turmoil, but we are not suggesting that we had any more trauma and stress than most other American families experience over time.

So what's the point in telling about everything we were going through in the years leading up to our diagnoses?

The point is this: *unrelenting stress that is not channeled through healthy outlets will make you sick.*

Had we had a healthy lifestyle in terms of nutrition, exercise and spiritual wellness, our bodies almost certainly would have been better able to cope with the stress. However, we lived almost entirely on fast food: pizza, burgers, chips, chocolate, and other assorted junk. If we thought about food at all, it was to wonder, *"Who has time to plan, shop for, and prepare nutritious meals when their lives are as out of control as ours?"*

We did not take vitamins or supplements (although I tried to remember to pop a children's chewable into the boys' mouths each morning).

We didn't drink alcohol in support of family members who struggled with that particular demon, but we didn't drink water, either. We drank tea, colas and coffee. In other words, we were dehydrated.

We had smoked for more than twenty years. (Seeing my parents' anguish during my brother's illness, I realized I couldn't watch them watch another of their children die, and I was the only one left. A few months after his death, I quit smoking, and Roger quit three days later.)

We operated on little (sometimes no) sleep.

We never exercised (who had time?) and we never took a vacation (who had that kind of money?). We couldn't afford to go out for meals or movies; entertainment of any kind was usually out of the question due to lack of money and time.

We both carried anger and resentment from unhappy first marriages, and I struggled with painful issues from my childhood.

And, while we believed in God and even talked about Him on holidays and special occasions, we didn't make time for Him in our daily lives.

Simply stated, our focus was just on getting through each day and wondering what the next day would bring. It never occurred to us that living this way was killing us.

But it was.

It is often said that stress kills. That's not exactly true. What stress *does* is lower our resistance to things that kill and our ability to fight them when they attack. When we live with chronic, unrelieved stress, our immune systems suffer the consequences. Our resistance to disease is lowered by poor nutrition and a sedentary lifestyle which are stressors in and of themselves. A sense that the future holds little hope leads to depression which further weakens our immune systems and gives us even less incentive to take care of ourselves, thus perpetuating the cycle.

It was no wonder we got sick. It's only a wonder it didn't happen sooner.

The first absolutely essential concept to understand when facing a diagnosis of cancer is that it is not one disease caused by one risk factor such as a genetic predisposition or smoking. There are more than one hundred types of cancer and, while many risk factors have been discovered, risk factors for some cancers are still mysteries to medical researchers.

You may be surprised to know that your body has been fighting cancer all your life! From time to time (possibly even every day, according to some experts), cells in your body have begun the abnormal division that can lead to cancer, but your healthy immune system kicked in and did its job, destroying the out-of-control cells and preventing the growth of tumors and spread of malignant cells.

The operative words in the above paragraph are *healthy immune system*. Cancer has to find a chink in your armor in order to take hold. Not all chinks can be prevented or repaired. After all, with any luck, most of us grow old (age is a risk factor for many cancers), and we can't change our genetic makeup or family medical history. But with a healthy lifestyle and emotional and spiritual well-being, most of the chinks can be prevented, and many of the existing ones can be repaired.

Cancer is just one of the many ways in which our bodies can be attacked when our immune systems are weakened by chronic, unrelieved stress. Heart disease is another. High blood pressure, frequent colds and infections… the list is endless.

We don't mean to suggest that *every* cancer, heart attack, stroke, virus or bacterial infection is the result of not taking care of oneself. After all, babies are born with cancer, marathon runners have heart attacks, nutrition experts get colds, doctors get infections, and great spiritual leaders have strokes.

But we can all reduce our risks of having to deal with these medical problems if we follow thoroughly researched and well-established guidelines for good health. What's more, by taking better care of ourselves physically, emotionally and spiritually, we can increase the odds of favorable outcomes when we do face life-threatening medical conditions.

Here's the baffling part: we knew those guidelines all along, and so do you. Why? Because Mom was right!

Mom didn't need the American Cancer Society or the American Heart Association to tell her how to raise a healthy family. How many of us grew up being told to eat our vegetables? How many of us were told to eat an apple instead of a cookie? How many times did she tell us to go to bed earlier, and how many times did she remind us to say our prayers? And how many times did Mom tell us to go outside and get some fresh air?

Speaking of fresh air, we wonder to this day whether an incident that occurred in our home about ten years before our diagnoses had anything to do with our cancers.

A termite inspection had revealed the destructive little pests were getting a hold on the foundation of our home. The exterminator's representative explained that his service person would drill holes under the foundation of the house and inject a pesticide into the holes and deep down into the soil. The termites would be exterminated, and there would be no pesticide odor inside the house.

"You'll never even know we were here," he reassured us.

Roger and the boys weren't home on the day the service was performed. I watched from the kitchen window as the worker disappeared under the house through a small door. Minutes later, I saw him stumble from beneath the house, pulling his protective suit off as he ran across the yard. As I watched in surprise, the house began to fill up with a powerful, sickening stench. In spite of the fact that the outside temperature was only twenty-eight degrees, I threw open the windows and doors, then ran out onto the front porch to breathe fresh air.

When the worker came back around to the front of the house, I asked him what had happened. He said the pesticide canister had "exploded" before its contents could be properly emptied and that he would have to go back to the shop for another canister. He assured me the fumes, while unpleasant, were not dangerous.

"Can't hurt you," he insisted. "I breathe them all the time."

I spent most of the day working around the house, taking frequent breaks to stand on the porch. The fumes were overwhelming, and I experienced bouts of nausea. By the time Roger and the boys came home, the house was pretty well aired out, but the lingering odor remained for several days.

About a week later, I awoke to an alarming symptom. My mouth had a slightly metallic taste, but I could not taste anything I ate or drank. During the next day or two, this strange symptom became worse. My mouth began to burn, and the metallic taste became stronger. Finally I went to the doctor.

He told me this was a classic symptom of exposure to a toxic chemical. I told him about the pesticide accident, and he said that almost certainly was the cause. He told me the bad news was there wasn't anything that could be done about it, but the good news was the condition would clear up on its own within a few months.

Although annoying, the metallic taste and the burning gradually disappeared, and my sense of taste returned a few months later. We chalked it up to a bad experience and forgot about it.

Until we were diagnosed with cancer and began to read articles about the connections between cancer and pesticides and other toxic chemicals.

There exists today a wealth of readily available information about environmental carcinogens and the risks of smoking, poor nutrition, lack of exercise, depression, stress and other factors that impact our physical, mental and emotional well-being. We can go online and download answers to whatever questions or concerns we have. We can find information about any subject that interests us in a matter of minutes. We can enter online chat rooms to give and receive support from others. We can call toll-free telephone lines for even more help.

But this information has been available for years in the more traditional formats of books and articles, not to mention all that advice from Mom.

So why haven't most of us been paying attention?

We believe there are two reasons.

The first is simply that we are human. We avoid unpleasant subjects whenever possible. We like to think we are immortal. We don't pay attention to things we don't want to hear until "life happens" and deals us a hard blow that forces us to listen.

The second is that medical professionals are trained in the diagnosis and treatment of conditions, diseases and injuries, but have little formal training in disease prevention. They are trained to write prescriptions. They are trained to perform surgeries. They are trained to read x-rays, set broken bones, cauterize wounds, and perform thousands of other medical procedures.

However, most doctors almost never talk to their patients about the lifestyle changes that can prevent disease and greatly improve quality and length of life for almost every human being.

Also, most of us live our lives with a cancer-is-something-that-happens-to-other-people-not-me mentality or the belief that only very old people get cancer. If you're reading this book, you have almost certainly discovered that those notions are untrue.

The bottom line then is that most of us *know* better, but we don't *do* better. And because our doctors don't write lifestyle changes on prescription blanks and insist that we make those changes, we just go along assuming that whatever goes wrong, the doctor can fix.

Until the day comes along – and it almost certainly will – when the doctor says, "I don't know if we can make you well or not, but we will do all that we can."

Before we go any further, we want to make sure you understand that we are not saying it is your "fault" if you have cancer. There is no fault here. You may have a genetic component that is exceptionally strong. An accident may have exposed you to toxic chemicals. Any number of factors beyond your control may have adversely affected your health.

But even if you have smoked all of your life, never exercised and eaten nothing but fast food and bon-bons, we're not trying to instill guilt here. Blame and guilt serve no purpose whatsoever.

However, knowledge *is* power! You have to understand how you got to where you are now in order to figure out how to turn around and go the other direction. You have to know what you were doing that may have contributed to your cancer so that you can stop doing it *now*. And you need to know what you were not doing before that you need to start doing *today*.

In retrospect, the notion that our unhealthy ways would someday catch up with us was probably always in the backs of our minds in the years leading up to our diagnoses. The mistake we made was in brushing it aside with the belief that we would be very old people before that happened. Never in our wildest nightmares did it occur to us that we would be the youngest married couple with a simultaneous diagnosis of cancer that most of our doctors had ever seen.

As we entered our forties – where so many insist that life begins – little did we know we were about to become a medical anomaly.

CHAPTER 2

Dark December

It's hard for us to believe now, but there really was a time in our lives when cancer had never been thought about or discussed, except perhaps in response to a news report of some famous person who had been diagnosed or a sad news item about a sick child. With the exception of my brother's illness and death, everyone in our family was relatively healthy, even the older members. Our friends were healthy. We didn't give much, if any, thought to cancer because it simply had never factored into our lives.

Back then we were just a mom and a dad doing the best we could to raise two teenage boys, make a decent living and deal with the day-to-day ups and downs of life. As mentioned earlier, our lives were stressful on many levels, but we didn't really think we had it any worse than anyone else.

Then the bottom fell out.

I had come in late on a December Friday after running errands all afternoon. Christmas was only ten days away and, in addition to the usual holiday craziness, we were also planning a party for Roger's employees and (along with his brothers and sister) a 50th wedding anniversary party for his parents. There was so much to do!

When I checked the answering machine, I heard Roger's voice. It seemed lower than usual and very controlled. Certainly not his usual cheerful self. The message said, "Please call me as soon as you get this."

Just the tone of his voice caused my hands to start shaking and my knees to feel weak. I knew something was wrong. Something *very* bad had happened.

I dialed his cell phone as quickly as my fingers could punch the numbers, and he answered on the first ring.

"What's wrong?" I blurted out.

"I need you to meet me at Dr. Reston's office as soon as you can. I'll wait for you out front."

What's wrong?" I asked again.

"I really don't know yet. He'll talk to us both when you get here."

I was trembling so badly I wondered if I would be able to drive. My stomach was in knots and my head was spinning with all the possibilities of what the news might be.

Roger had been seeing Dr. Reston for what we all assumed was a urinary tract infection. Several weeks earlier, Roger had experienced a brief, sharp pain in his side when he urinated and had passed a small bit of blood. He told me about it, and I insisted he go to the doctor. At first he refused, saying it had only happened that one time and he felt fine, but I finally persuaded him to see a urologist.

Dr. Reston had ordered some tests, but stated from the outset that it was probably just a urinary tract infection. When the results had come back from an x-ray a few days before, he had asked Roger if he knew he only had one kidney.

Roger was stunned, of course. He had never even heard of such a thing. The doctor said it was an unusual condition, but not a troubling one. He had seen it before, he said, but patients with the condition almost never know they have it until a problem arises requiring an x-ray. He had shown Roger the x-ray and, indeed, only one kidney could be seen.

While this information had taken a little while for us to process, we had agreed to "put it on our list of things not to worry about" (Roger's list, not mine!) because the doctor had assured us his other kidney was healthy and had apparently been doing the work of two for more than forty years.

In the meantime, though, Dr. Reston had ordered a CT scan "just to cover all the bases." This time, the doctor was in for an even bigger shock, as were we all.

This was the reason we had been called to his office.

When I pulled into the parking lot at the medical center, Roger was pacing up and down the sidewalk. Before I could get out of the car, he got in. He was pale and shaking, and he laid his head on my shoulder and began to cry. I wrapped my arms around him and pulled him close and tight as he whispered, "I think I have cancer."

I don't remember what I thought or said next. I only remember a sense of disbelief and confusion, a momentary certainty that I had heard wrong.

The next thing I remember thinking – and it must have been several minutes later – was that we needed to get inside and hear what the doctor had to say. Surely Roger was wrong. Surely he had misunderstood something in their brief telephone conversation, and we needed to hear from the doctor as soon as possible that this was all a mistake.

Dr. Reston took us into his private office, and we sat on an expensive-looking leather couch. It's true that when you are in shock, your world sort of goes into slow motion and every detail becomes excruciatingly clear and suspended in time. I will remember forever the rich color and feel of that couch and the way the sunlight entered the office through the blinds, low and at a slight angle because of the season and the time of day. I remember hearing the water fountain humming in the hallway outside the door. And I remember seeing all the diplomas and certificates on the walls of the office and thinking *surely this learned, skilled man can fix whatever is wrong!*

The doctor began. "Roger, you have a ten-centimeter tumor in your right kidney. It is completely filling the kidney which is why that kidney didn't show up on the x-rays. The CT scan showed us that the kidney is indeed there, but it is filled with this very large tumor."

I thought, *O.K., this is good. He hasn't said "cancer." He's only said "tumor."*

Roger must have been thinking the same thing. He said, "So now you do a biopsy to see if it's malignant or not, right?"

"No. Tumors in the kidney are almost always malignant. It's a pretty sure bet that this one is."

Skipped heartbeats. The sunlight. The humming water fountain. Certificates and diplomas. I willed everything to freeze right then and there. *No more*, I thought. *Everybody stop! Don't say anything else!*

"Am I going to die?" Roger whispered.

The doctor shrugged. "I've had patients with much smaller tumors who died and patients with larger tumors who survived. I'd say it's fifty-fifty."

He said it so matter-of-factly. Had he forgotten he was talking to a patient and his wife? Why was he speaking to us like we were medical colleagues discussing a case in a textbook?

Fifty-fifty. Roger might die. Or he might not.

Dr. Reston began to explain what lay ahead. Because the kidney is made up almost entirely of blood vessels, and because Roger's tumor was so large, the kidney itself would have to be removed. To remove the kidney, a rib would also be removed. The doctor would not know whether the malignancy had spread until the operation was well under-way, so he couldn't tell us at this time how extensive the surgery might be. But he made it clear that this was very major surgery. We could plan on Roger's being in the hospital for a week to ten days, followed by a recovery period at home of six to eight weeks.

"What about chemotherapy? Radiation? What else will we do?" one of us asked.

"There is no chemotherapy or radiation treatment for this type of cancer."

No chemotherapy. No radiation. We knew so little about cancer that we didn't even know there are cancers for which there is no treatment other than surgery or even that different cancers respond better to some treatments than others. We knew virtually nothing about cancer except that the word itself was frightening to say because of its deadly implications. Wasn't that the reason many people referred to it as "The Big 'C'"?

"You mean you either get it all with surgery or you don't?" Roger asked.

"That's pretty much it. If we get in there and find that the tumor is completely contained within the kidney and there is no evidence of metastasis, the prognosis will be pretty good. If we find there is lymph node involvement or other metastasis, the prognosis will not be so good. Renal cell carcinoma is a very slow-growing type of cancer. Considering the size of your tumor, it's possible you have had it for as many as ten years, and that increases the likelihood of metastasis. We just won't know until we go in and see what we're dealing with."

Ten years! To say we were in shock would be the all-time under-statement. I thought briefly of the pesticide incident ten years earlier, but how could someone have cancer for ten years and not know? How could there have been no symptoms?

And what were those other words he had used? Metastasis? Renal cell what? Carcinoma? And what were lymph nodes?

We were numb. It felt like the world had stopped going around, thrown us off and started up again without us.

The doctor continued to talk. We participated as much as we could in the discussion regarding the scheduling of the surgery. Dr. Reston wanted to perform the surgery immediately, but Roger insisted it would have to wait until after Christmas. After all, he reasoned, if the tumor had been there for as many as ten years, what difference would a couple of weeks make?

Dr. Reston scheduled the surgery for December 28. He said he would need the assistance of another surgeon and that the procedure would be four to five hours long barring unforeseen complications. He told us other details, but we only partially heard him. He said he wanted to see us again on Monday after he had had time to consult with the surgeon who would assist him.

The doctor then said he would leave us alone for a while, and he left the room.

It was all I could do to keep from jumping up and running out of the building. Amazingly, Roger was already going into his "okay-here's-what-we-do-now" mode. He immediately said we were not going to tell anyone about this until after the holidays. True to the generous heart and spirit I had fallen in love with thirteen years earlier, Roger's first thoughts were for everyone else.

"We are not going to ruin Christmas for everyone," he said. "And we are not going to spoil my parents' anniversary. After the holidays, we'll tell whoever needs to know."

I just nodded my head, not knowing how we could keep those who love us the most from knowing. Wouldn't they see in our faces that something was desperately, terribly wrong?

Then I realized I would have to tell my own parents. We would need them to help us take care of the boys during Roger's hospitalization, I told him, and it wouldn't be fair to the children or my parents to spring it on them at the last minute. Some plans just had to be made right then.

Roger finally agreed. We pulled ourselves together as much as possible and left the doctor's office.

My memory of the rest of that evening is fuzzy. It had gotten late, and it was dark and very cold. I don't remember driving at all, but I must have because Roger and I were in separate cars.

Then somehow we were with my parents and our boys. We told them everything, but slanted the information enough to convince Ryan and Reid there was nothing to worry about. Dad would be fine. He was just going to have to have a "*really big* operation" after Christmas and wouldn't be up and around for a while. This was enough for them to deal with at the time, we thought, and they were fine with the explanation.

My parents offered to take the boys home with them overnight. Ryan and Reid jumped at the chance because staying with their grandparents meant staying up as late as they liked and generally being spoiled. Our reaction was *Good. They're behaving normally. This has all gone right over their heads.*

We went home and spent the entire weekend alternating between tears and stunned silence. We abandoned our favorite chairs in the living room to sit next to one another on the couch, holding hands, stroking arms, each of us trying desperately to ease our own and the other's pain. If one of us left the room for even a minute, the other one called out, "Are you okay?" The one who had left always answered, "Yes, I'm fine."

What a lie. We were far from fine. That weekend we learned what chilling, knee-buckling terror is.

That weekend we also made a pact with one another that we would never again see a doctor on a Friday. As the hours went by and the shock wore off, we thought of a hundred questions. What causes kidney cancer? Will Roger need a blood transfusion during surgery? How will his pain be controlled? What do we need to do at home to help him recover? How and when will the doctors know if they got all the cancer? With the weekend looming ahead, there was no one to answer our questions. Little did we know it then but, just by thinking of these questions, we were already learning valuable cancer survival tools.

In the back of my mind were the truly horrible questions, the ones I didn't dare say out loud. *What if they don't get it all? How can I possibly live if he doesn't?*

Somehow we made it to Monday. We met with Dr. Reston again. He answered many of our questions and gave us a more in-depth explanation of the surgery and recovery period.

During that visit, Roger said to him, "I'm going to be the best patient you've ever had." I knew that was his way of saying *I am putting my life in your hands. Please don't let me die.*

We gritted our teeth and smiled through the days that followed, through the business and family holiday parties and Roger's parents' anniversary dinner. On one hand, we wanted time to stand still so we wouldn't have to move forward into the dark unknown. To that extent, we made a point of being exceptionally aware of every encounter with friend or relative. We held people closer and hugged them longer. We savored every morsel of holiday fare. We hung on every note of every Christmas carol and took painstaking care with every decorating detail.

We wanted to stretch out each happy moment and pleasurable sensation because the reality was that this might be our last Christmas as a complete family. (We were learning more valuable cancer survival tools, but we still didn't know it!)

On the other hand, we wanted this terrible thing in Roger's body to be out as soon as possible.

We broke the news to Roger's family the day after Christmas. His sister Mary, a surgical nurse, helped their parents understand the diagnosis, but she and we tried to downplay the danger for their sake. We tried to be upbeat and acted as if we were sure everything would turn out fine.

As a Christmas gift, I had given Roger a theatre package that included a romantic dinner at an upscale restaurant in a nearby city, a trolley ride to the theatre to see a touring production of *The Phantom of the Opera*, and a luxury hotel suite for the night.

So on the twenty-sixth of December, Ryan and Reid enjoyed another night of spoiling by their grandparents, and we went off to dinner and the theatre. We agreed beforehand not to talk about what lay less than forty-eight hours ahead, and we both made a good show of enjoying dinner and the musical. But both of us were thinking and fearing the worst – that this might be our last romantic night together, if not forever, then at least for a very long time.

The last words Roger said that night as we lay in the dark in each other's arms were, "I'm scared."

I replied, "Me, too."

We arrived at the hospital on the morning of the twenty-eighth at some ungodly hour before dawn. We were taken to a third-floor room where nurses and technicians began prepping Roger for surgery. We kept up a cheerful but nervous banter with them.

Then, to my utter dismay, Roger began cracking jokes. Now, granted, he had always had a wonderfully wicked sense of humor, but I couldn't believe my ears when he started joking with the medical personnel who were poking him and doing all manner of uncomfortable and unpleasant procedures to his body as if he were a rag doll.

When a plastic band with his blood type was placed on his arm, he asked the nurse, "Does this mean we're engaged?" When another nurse asked him what type of surgery he was having, he explained that he had renal cell carcinoma and the surgeon would be removing his right kidney. She said, "I'm really sorry." He looked down sadly, grimaced and said, "Yeah. Me, too. That's my favorite kidney." We all laughed out loud.

Roger's jokes kept everyone's spirits up. For as long as he was in the room, I was able to smile and laugh.

Then the gurney arrived to take him to surgery. I walked beside the gurney to the elevator, then leaned to kiss him. We exchanged "I love you's." I smiled and waved as the elevator doors closed, then dissolved into tears in the comforting arms of a nurse.

Soon Mary and my mother arrived, and the three of us tried to comfort and reassure one another during the four-and-a-half hour wait. The longest hours must surely be those spent in hospital waiting rooms (although chemotherapy hours may be tied for this distinction).

When Dr. Reston entered the room, we rushed to meet him. He said the surgery was over and it had gone well. Roger was in the recovery room, and I would be called as soon as he was taken to the "Step-Down Unit" (so called because it is a level of care one step down from Intensive Care). The doctor said many things, but the only words I heard were, "We're pretty sure we got it all." I knew that whatever else he said and whatever medical jargon confused his message, Mary would explain it to me later. For now, all that mattered was that Roger was out of surgery and the prognosis was generally optimistic.

Several more hours passed before I was called to the Step-Down Unit. Mom and Mary left as only one family member per patient was allowed on the unit.

I was waiting at the door of the SDU before Roger was transported there from the recovery room. When a gurney was wheeled past me and turned into the unit, I looked at the unconscious patient on it and wondered when Roger would be brought here. A nurse said to me, "Mrs. Cawthon, please wait out here until we have Mr. Cawthon settled. Then you can come in and see him." The patient on the gurney was my own husband, and I had not recognized him!

His head and neck were wrapped in warming towels and blankets. Only his face was visible, and it was swollen beyond recognition. An oxygen mask covered his nose and mouth. Tubes emerged from under the blankets at various locations up and down the length of the gurney only to disappear at some other place further on. Monitors beeped and clicked all around. His arms and hands were shaking beneath the covers.

I was dumbfounded. I had never seen anyone so ill. It was almost impossible to believe this was the same man who, only hours before, had had all the nurses on the third floor laughing.

After he was settled, Roger's eyes opened briefly and he appeared to be fighting the oxygen mask. Afraid to touch him, I summoned the nurse. She removed the mask, satisfied herself that he no longer needed it, and put it away. He seemed relieved and closed his eyes again.

Just before the surgery, Roger had been made to remove the only jewelry he ever wore, his West Point ring and his wedding ring. I had been holding them for him. Now I leaned down, kissed him on the cheek and slipped his wedding ring back where it belonged. His eyes opened at my touch, and he whispered hoarsely, "Will you marry me?"

He was still making jokes. It was a good sign.

The Step-Down Unit had four patients and two nurses in the room at all times. According to the posted rules of the unit, each patient's one family member was allowed a ten-minute visit every hour. But I never moved from Roger's bedside, and no one ever told me to.

He drifted in and out of consciousness all that afternoon and evening, rousing briefly from time to time to press the button in his hand that administered morphine for the pain. I watched him sleep, watched the nurses check him periodically, watched and waited.

Late that evening, a tall man in a suit came into the room, picked up Roger's chart, read it and began to examine him. I had never seen him before.

"I'm Roger's wife," I said. "Who are you?"

He apparently had not seen me sitting there in the shadows of the dimly lit room.

"I'm sorry," he said, then introduced himself. "I was the anesthesiologist during your husband's surgery this morning. I'm glad to see he's stable. He sure gave us a scare."

Puzzled, I asked him to explain. Dr. Nelson told me that Roger had begun to lose so much blood during the surgery that he had turned the anesthesiology duties over to a nurse anesthetist so that he could assist the two surgeons in bringing the bleeding under control. Dr. Nelson revealed the shocking fact that Roger had lost eight pints of blood during the operation.

"He was bleeding it out faster than we could put it back in. It took three of us to get it under control. It was really touch-and-go there for awhile."

I realized then that something had been nagging at the back of my mind all day, something I hadn't been able to put my finger on. Now I knew what it was. When Dr. Reston had come to the waiting room to tell us how the surgery had gone, my subconscious had registered how fresh and clean he looked. His surgical scrubs were spotless and looked freshly ironed. Now I understood why. There had been a great deal of blood. It must have been everywhere. Dr. Reston had changed into clean scrubs before talking to his patient's family.

Three days in the Step-Down Unit passed slowly. Roger remained unconscious for the most part, only occasionally waking enough to push the morphine button before drifting off again.

I was amazed to see his incision for the first time. He had been cut almost completely in half, from the middle of his back all the way around to the middle of his abdomen. Fifty-six surgical staples held the huge incision closed.

On the fourth day, a semi-conscious Roger was moved to a private room. I learned quickly that the surgical floor was operating with a "skeleton staff" (horrible term!) as many medical personnel had taken vacation days during the holiday season. The floor was precariously understaffed, and the nurses were overworked to the point of exhaustion.

Once the nursing staff saw that Roger had a family member present all the time, they entered the room only to check and record his vital signs and provide minimal nursing care.

He began a roller-coaster ride of fevers, sweats and chills as his body fought to stave off infection. One minute he was burning up, and the next minute he was shivering and his teeth were chattering. With each episode, his hospital gown and the bed sheets were soaked, yet no one came to bathe him or change the linens. My sister-in-law Mary helped me bathe him and change his gown, and together we changed the bedding.

Roger began to wake up on the sixth day following his surgery, and was fully alert by the eighth day. By day nine he was beginning to complain about the hospital food and fuss to go home, always a sign that a patient is taking his first steps on the road to recovery.

We finally left the hospital on the tenth day. There was nothing to do now but wait and see if the cancer would resurface. We were told it could show up in Roger's lungs, his bones, his liver, his brain. If it did, the prognosis would be grim.

These were dark days, but they would soon turn even darker.

CHAPTER 3

The Red Devil...

The first months of 1996 were cold and bleak, but the days began to grow a little brighter inside our house. Roger was recovering rapidly from his surgery. He was eager to bathe and dress himself and to come downstairs for meals with the family. He was a cheerful patient and never complained of pain or discomfort. He rested when he needed to rest, and he pushed himself when he needed to push.

He believed with all his heart that he was well, that Dr. Reston had indeed "gotten it all." I wanted to believe, and even pretended to believe, but I was still terrified the cancer would reappear somewhere else in Roger's body. His good spirits were contagious, though, and as January turned into February, I began to relax somewhat and tried hard to believe that everything really would be okay.

Sunday morning, February 11, was sunny, but bitterly cold. I planned to fix our usual big Sunday breakfast for my husband and sons, and Roger wanted to get dressed and come downstairs to eat. He refused my help, so while he labored to dress himself, I took a shower.

As I spread the rich, soapy lather over my chest, my right hand froze on the far side of my left breast. There was a hard lump just beneath the skin. My fingers traced its outline. It was nearly the size of a golf ball.

Despite the warm water pouring over me, my blood ran cold. I tasted terror in the back of my throat, and my heart hammered against my ribcage. My knees trembled, and I stumbled and nearly fell getting out of the shower. Clutching a towel around me, I ran into the bedroom and choked out the words, "What is this? *What is this?*"

Roger gently touched the lump with his fingers. I saw the light go out of his eyes, his mouth become grim. He said simply, "I don't know, but it can't be what you're thinking. It can't be. There's just no way."

I nodded and repeated what he'd said, wanting to believe it. "You're right. It couldn't be."

But I didn't believe it, and I don't think he did either. I spent the rest of that day fighting panic as Roger tried to reassure both himself and me.

I had been faithful in getting my annual mammograms for many years and had, in fact, had one only nine months earlier. It had not indicated any areas of concern. I had also had a clinical exam that included a breast exam by our family physician only six months earlier. He had not found anything either.

I had never, however, performed a thorough breast self-exam (BSE), which the American Cancer Society advocates for women beginning as early as age twenty. On a hit-and-miss basis, I had occasionally found a hardened area in one of my breasts when showering, but it always disappeared in a week or so. When I discussed these with my doctor, he said they were probably cysts (which are almost always benign) and that I should cut back on foods and drinks containing caffeine.

He also told me that I had very dense breast tissue and that most young women do. This is why younger women's breasts are firmer and higher up – "perkier," if you will! – than older women's. As estrogen production decreases in later years, breast tissue becomes less dense, and breasts begin to lose their firmness.

What he did not tell me – and what no one had ever told me – was that this density of the breast tissue in younger women makes interpreting their mammograms and clinical breast exams more difficult for physicians and thus less reliable than those same tests performed on older patients.

I was on the phone with the clinic where I have my mammograms performed as soon as they opened Monday morning. I tried to sound calm, but my voice and hands were shaking.

"I need to schedule a mammogram," I told the receptionist.

She pulled my file and said, "I'm sorry, Mrs. Cawthon, but it has only been nine months since your last mammogram. Your insurance won't pay for another one until it has been a year."

"I don't care if I have to pay for it," I said. Then I began to break down. "I have a lump in my left breast. It's big and it's hard, and I'm scared."

She told me to come right in.

The mammogram was performed that very morning, and I was told the radiologist would call me later that afternoon if he thought there was any cause for concern. I went home to wait.

The dreaded phone call came late in the day.

"You need to schedule an appointment with your surgeon," Dr. O'Donald told me.

"Do I have cancer?" I blurted out.

"There is really no way to say for sure from a mammogram," he said, but I could tell he wasn't saying everything he was thinking. I persisted.

"Do you *think* it might be cancer?" I demanded.

There was silence for a moment. Then he said quietly, "Yes, I think it probably is. You need to schedule an appointment with your surgeon."

My knees were so weak I could no longer stand. I sank to the floor, the phone still in my hand. I managed to explain that I didn't have a surgeon (the surgeon who had performed Roger's surgery was a urologist), but that I would find one. He said to have the surgeon call his office so that my x-rays could be forwarded.

My memory of the rest of that week is a blur. Mary recommended a new young surgeon at the hospital where she worked. She said Dr. Blevins was so good that other doctors and surgeons were going to him for their own surgeries and sending family members and friends to him, too.

On Wednesday I was in Dr. Blevins' office. He looked like a teenager, but his manner was so professional and reassuring that I immediately felt comfortable with him and confident in his skill and expertise.

After examining me, making some notations about the lump, and asking questions about my medical history, he said there was a very good chance the lump would prove to be a benign tumor or hardened cyst. Therefore he would remove only the lump and some surrounding tissue. If the biopsy showed the tissue to be malignant, we would make further decisions down the line.

On Friday morning I was in surgery, and on Friday afternoon I was home.

We waited eight agonizing days for the results of the biopsy as the doctor was out of town; it was his policy not to let anyone else give his patients biopsy results.

Roger and I went together to Dr. Blevins' office to learn the results.

The doctor entered the examining room and opened my file. He said, "I'm sorry to tell you, but the results of the biopsy were positive for breast cancer."

I started to shake, and a low moan came up from somewhere deep inside me. A nurse ran to get me a cup of water, but my hands trembled so much when I took it that water splashed everywhere.

Roger was choking back tears as he said to the doctor, "I don't believe this. We *both* have cancer!"

The doctor shook his head and said, "I know. I'd heard. It is pretty hard to believe, and I'm so sorry."

He waited for us to calm down a bit before he continued.

"There is some good news. The pathologist's report says we got clean margins, meaning we took sufficient tissue around the tumor to ensure we got every bit of it. Also, the type of breast cancer you have is a very non-aggressive type."

Type? I never knew there were "types" of breast cancer. I thought breast cancer was breast cancer.

He continued. "What we need to do now is remove some of the lymph nodes underneath your arm just to be sure there is no spread of the cancer. I'm almost completely certain there is not since the tumor margins were clean, but it's a necessary precaution. If the lymph nodes are not involved, you will probably only need to have some radiation treatments. I don't think we're looking at anything more than that right now."

Clean margins. Non-aggressive. No chemotherapy. Those were all good things, I figured, but I was still in shock, numb and limp as a dishrag. I learned that day that fear has peaks and valleys. Intense fear can only be sustained for so long before it plummets, leaving you weak and exhausted and oddly calm.

I remained in that state until my next surgery several days later. This time I spent the night in the hospital. During the surgery, a drainage tube had been inserted under my arm to remove the lymph fluid that builds up after the removal of lymph nodes. I went home the next day after a nurse instructed me in emptying the plastic bladder that filled with fluid several times a day. I remember thinking it looked like a hand grenade.

Once again, we waited more than a week to learn the results of the biopsy. And once again, the doctor was as dumbfounded as we were by the report. Ironically, the date was March 15, the anniversary of my brother's death, the infamous Ides of March about which my brother and I had often joked.

"We removed sixteen lymph nodes," Dr. Blevins told us. "Four of them were positive for cancer. I was so surprised that I drove over to the hospital to see the slides for myself."

This time, Roger just wrapped his arms around me and we were silent.

There was more bad news. Some of the cells that had spread to my lymph nodes were of the non-aggressive type of breast cancer that had turned up in the original biopsy, but some were of a much more aggressive type of breast cancer. Basically, I had two types of breast cancer.

At this point, Dr. Blevins said he would be consulting with an oncologist to determine the next step, and that I would be hearing from the oncologist's office.

The drainage tube had been removed by this time, and I continued to see Dr. Blevins every few days to have the fluid that continued to build up removed. A large needle attached to a pump was used for this, but there was no pain. I was beginning to learn some of the long-term effects of my surgeries. Nerves had been severed, and places along the inside of my arm and beneath it probably would remain numb forever.

The worst part of this entire period was that no one talked to us about what the implications of my diagnosis were. No one gave us any literature to read, no one offered me the phone number of a support network to call, no one gave me the name of a contact person to talk to. We knew nothing about breast cancer, and no one offered us any information or support.

Until the phone rang early one Monday morning more than a month after my first surgery. It was a nurse at an oncologist's office and she was calling to schedule an appointment for me with a doctor I had never heard of, but who would come to be one of the most influential and important people in my life.

Roger went with me to see Dr. Mason. Roger and I went everywhere together now. We were each other's lifelines. Each of us was the only one who could really understand what the other was going through. His recovery from his surgery was progressing well, but he was far from being considered cured of cancer. Now we feared for both of our lives. It was so far-fetched and so unthinkable that at times I truly believed it must be a bad dream.

In fact, for two relatively young people married to each other to have simultaneous cancer diagnoses was such an unusual occurrence that Dr. Mason told us during our first meeting with him that we had had a "better chance of winning the lottery." He said he had seen simultaneous diagnoses of both a husband and wife with cancer in much older couples, couples in their 70s, 80s and 90s. But it was practically unheard of in a couple our age.

Dr. Mason spent two hours with us that day. He pulled a chair up close and talked to us eye-to-eye. And when I asked him if I was going to die, he said the most remarkable thing.

"Sure you are! We all are! But you're not going to die today or tomorrow or next week or next year if I can help it."

I felt hope for the first time in weeks as he continued. "You need a course of chemotherapy, and then you will need a series of radiation treatments. I won't lie to you. It's not going to be easy, but if you will do everything I tell you to do, I believe you will look back on this one day and it will seem like it happened to someone else."

He went over the details of my diagnosis with us and explained that an important report still had not come in. That report would be from a lab 3,000 miles away in California! A specimen from my tumor had been sent to that lab to determine whether I was a candidate for an oral drug known as Tamoxifen, which, at that time, was considered the best defense against a recurrence of certain breast cancers.

We also discussed Roger's case with Dr. Mason that day. Roger had never been referred to an oncologist as we had been told there was no course of treatment for him other than surgery, and we still knew next to nothing about renal cell carcinoma. But Dr. Mason reassured us that, while Roger's cancer was a "particularly nasty one," there were other treatment options to be considered if the cancer reappeared.

In the weeks before this meeting, I had lost ten or fifteen pounds because I had been too nervous and upset to eat. I had hardly slept at all, and what sleep I had was not restful. Dr. Mason wrote a prescription for a mild sedative.

He called the next day to tell me the report was in from the lab in California. It indicated I was a candidate for Tamoxifen.

I said, "That's a good thing, right? It gives us one more weapon to use, doesn't it?"

He agreed. Then he said, "You sound like you're feeling better today."

"The medication you prescribed is wonderful. I had a good night's sleep, and I've eaten today. Thank you so much."

I realize now that those first two hours spent with Dr. Mason were the beginning of a new me and a new Roger. Our dual diagnosis of cancer was the end of the life we had known before. This was the start of a journey that would lead us to know our real selves for the first time and to reevaluate everything we had ever thought we knew about living.

We met with Dr. Mason again several days later. This time he went over my course of treatment with us. I would have four treatments ("cycles") of a combination of the powerful cancer drugs Adriamycin and Cytoxin. Adriamycin, he told me, is sometimes called the "Red Devil" or "Red Death." It looks like red Kool-Aid, and it is one of the chemotherapy drugs that causes nausea and vomiting in many patients. He explained that this drug had been in use for many years and that long ago, before the correct dosages had been determined, patients had sometimes been cured of their cancer only to die of heart failure because Adriamycin can destroy a small percentage of the heart muscle. It is also the drug that causes many patients to lose their hair. This information was so unnerving that I don't recall anything he said about the other drug.

Dr. Mason then asked if I would like to participate in a clinical trial. I had never heard the term. He explained that I was a good candidate for a research study of a drug known as Taxol. The trial was currently entering its final phase, which meant the drug had already proven to be a powerful weapon in the war on breast cancer and now needed only some fine-tuning in terms of dosage. If I agreed, my name would be entered into a computer. The computer would randomly select patients to be in the experimental group (those who would receive Taxol) and patients to be in the control group (those who would not receive Taxol, but who would still receive the standard course of treatment). If the computer selected me for the experimental group, the trial would add four more cycles of chemotherapy to my treatment plan.

As frightening as all of this was, I remember thinking that I wanted every weapon I could possibly get to fight this battle. I was scared of the treatments and their side effects, but I was more scared of not getting well. I agreed to the clinical trial.

Dr. Mason then introduced me to a study nurse who would oversee my treatment since I had agreed to the clinical trial. She handed me a thirteen-page consent form, told me to read it and initial each page at the bottom. Then she left the room.

We couldn't believe what we read in those thirteen pages! They outlined every possible side effect of treatment including "thrombotic events" (strokes), seizures and heart attacks. Roger kept saying things like, "They just have to put that in to cover their butts if it happens" and "I'll bet that's only happened once, but they have to put it in there for legal reasons." I initialed each page.

When the nurse came back, she handed me a sheet of paper with six monthly calendars on it. They were labeled March through August, and each one contained numerous notations of appointments and tests. I'd never seen anything like it! Before I could begin my chemotherapy, I had to have a chest x-ray, cardiac sonogram, bone scan and a variety of other tests to get "baseline" readings (for the purpose of later comparison) and to determine that I was strong enough to withstand the rigors of treatment. I even had to schedule check-ups with my dentist, eye doctor, dermatologist and gynecologist.

The chemotherapy cycles would be three weeks apart, but there were appointments in-between for blood work and other tests to determine how I was tolerating the treatments. She gave me a small book I was to bring with me each time so the nurses could record the results of my blood work. I guess it was to give me a kind of visual reading of how I was progressing, which days between treatments were my weakest or sickest and on which days I began to recover.

I would begin taking Tamoxifen the day of my first chemotherapy treatment, and there were handfuls of other pills to take for the next six months. The purpose of most of them was to minimize or eliminate some of the more unpleasant side effects of treatment. I would also continue to take the sedative to help me sleep and stimulate my appetite; it would also be helpful in alleviating nausea.

Looking at the page of calendars with all of my appointments, I felt overwhelmed by what lay ahead. It was more than I could even comprehend. My eyes brimming with tears, I asked Roger, "How am I going to get through all of this?"

And he said the words that have become my mantra ever since. He said, "We're just going to show up one day at a time."

CHAPTER 4

...And an Angel in White

It is said that a journey of a thousand miles begins with a single step. And so it began.

I had my first chemotherapy treatment near the end of March, 1996. At the oncology clinic where Dr. Mason practiced, most patients received their chemotherapy treatments in a communal room. A dozen or so big recliner chairs with pillows and blankets were arranged in a semi-circle. Patients hooked up to tubes and pumps occupied most of the chairs on my first morning there. Nurses checked each patient periodically, chatting and doing what they could to make them comfortable. I was surprised to see the patients reading, listening to tapes, working crossword puzzles, knitting and chatting with each other. I was far too nervous to imagine doing any of those things, but I found it reassuring to think I might be able to some day.

I actually tolerated that first treatment pretty well. I experienced some nausea three or four days later, but it was not intolerable. I was pleasantly surprised and began to think this might not be as bad as I had anticipated. The dark cloud that had hung over me for months began to lift, and I began to believe that I would, indeed, look back on this one day and think it had happened to someone else.

Then I had my second treatment. And then my third. Chemotherapy can have a cumulative effect, and subsequent cycles were much harder to bounce back from than the first. After my third treatment, I was severely and almost constantly nauseated. The most innocuous aromas assaulted my sense of smell: hairspray, deodorant, soap, shampoo, perfume. I couldn't be within a hundred feet of anyone who smelled of any of these things. I asked my mother to stop wearing hairspray and Roger to switch to an unscented deodorant.

About this time, a "central line" was surgically implanted in my chest because my small veins had stopped cooperating, making it difficult for the nurses (and painful for me!) to administer my treatments and to draw blood.

Cancer, it's been said, is not for sissies. Besides the nausea, hair loss and pain, there are other side effects of treatment and little "surprises" that can and do sneak up on you and just flat kick your backside. There are no rules, and cancer never fights fair. Every case is different, every treatment is different, every outcome is different and every patient's experience is different.

For me, the other little "surprises" along the way included the loss of my eyelashes, eyebrows and, yes, every hair on my body. No one had told me that might happen. I even gained weight instead of losing it as I had thought I would. Round and bald, my body began to resemble that of a huge newborn baby. Before my chemotherapy was over, I was taking drugs to counteract the side effects of other drugs.

Exhausted and depressed, I sometimes felt I had left this world and was living in another one. Most of the time, I was quiet and listless. I had no fighting spirit left. I cried every day, sometimes from depression and despair, sometimes from the physical discomforts.

My illness and depression were taking a toll on Roger and our sons as well. Fears that his cancer would recur, a feeling of helplessness in the face of my misery, and the very real financial problems that were beginning to arise had taken the wind out of Roger's normally inflated sails.

Ryan and Reid had become distant and uncommunicative. We were all too aware of the changes in them, but we were too exhausted and sick to know what to do about it. My parents tried to help, often inviting the boys to spend the weekend, taking them fishing and on other outings. These escapes from home helped somewhat, but we could see in our sons' eyes that they thought they were losing both their mom and dad. And they didn't even know how to talk about it.

Our family was in anguish, spiraling downward emotionally, physically, and financially.

Efforts of relatives and friends to bring meals and offer comfort were well intentioned, but usually fell flat. The smell of rich casseroles sent me running to the bathroom. A hug from anyone wearing hair spray, perfume or scented deodorant caused me to gag. And when visitors told me how important it was for me to "keep a positive attitude," I smiled to their faces, but silently seethed.

Positive attitude? You have got to be kidding. My brother is dead, and now my family is watching me die. They won't say it, but I know that's what they're thinking. Do you know what I see every time I look in my mother's eyes? I can see she's thinking, "Oh, dear God, I'm losing my other child." Seeing that look on her face is more painful to me than any treatment I have been through.

My husband lost a kidney to cancer. If one little cancer cell escaped that surgery and sets up shop somewhere else in his body, he'll die. And then where will we all be? I will die without him, and then what will happen to the kids…oh, my God…

And look at me. I don't have a hair anywhere on my body. My eyebrows and eyelashes are gone. My eyes burn because my tear ducts have dried up. My nose and mouth are full of sores. I have a tube going into my chest so they can pump poison into my body every week. They tell me that every one of the chemotherapy drugs I'm taking can cause other cancers. And after the chemo treatments are finished, I get to go to the hospital every day for five weeks and get fried by radiation.

When I look in the mirror, I don't even know who that person is anymore. She's not me. She's some sad, sick woman who might get well, and who might not. And if she does, she gets to spend the rest of her life wondering when it's going to come back and when she's going to get to go through this all over again and how bad will it be next time and will the cancer kill me or will the damned treatments kill me first?

Positive attitude? Oh, please. How dare you? You don't even have a clue.

Even though I never voiced my bitter feelings, I must have worn them on my sleeve because visitors came less often. Finally, only my mother came to see me every day. She tried to keep our crumbling family together. She attempted to discipline the boys and help them understand what we were all going through, and she tried mightily to get them to open up and talk about what *they* were going through. Ryan and Reid, though, just stayed gone as much as possible. Who could blame them? There was nothing in our house but an atmosphere of illness and despair.

My mother fixed meals for the family, cleaned the house and did the laundry. Sometimes she just crawled into bed next to me and held me.

Throughout the months of treatment, I often took out and unfolded the piece of paper with my treatment schedule on it. I faithfully crossed out every day, every treatment, every blood test, every visit with the doctor. This small act became a ritual, the numbers on the calendars my prayer beads.

My lowest point occurred about halfway through my five months of chemotherapy treatments. I awoke one morning believing I would die that day and actually taking some relief from that thought. It would be okay because I just couldn't imagine feeling that sick any longer. I didn't see how anyone could feel that sick and *not* die.

My insides felt like they were cooking. The nausea was unbearable. I didn't have enough strength to dress myself.

My mother – who had taken on the full burden of my care so Roger could go back to work – dressed me and drove me to the oncology clinic.

After examining me, Dr. Mason ordered IV fluids and some other medications as I was severely dehydrated. I was placed on a bed in a private room, and a nurse started the IV. She told me she would be back to check on me, and then left the room.

What happened next is quite literally the most amazing thing that has ever happened to me. It defies worldly explanation, and it taught me the most valuable lesson I have learned in this life.

Alone on the bed in that room, watching the clear fluid drip through the tube leading to my chest, I surrendered. I told God that I was too tired and sick to fight anymore. Believing I was dying, I prayed that my children, husband, parents and anyone else who cared about me be comforted. That was all I wanted, and it was all that mattered.

Some time later, another nurse came into the room. She smiled at me as she checked the IV drip and arranged the covers around me.

"Hi!" she said cheerfully. "I'm Susan. Heard you're having a rough day."

"I think I'm going to die today," I murmured.

Susan pulled a chair next to the bed and sat down. She took my hand in one of hers and began to gently stroke my arm with her other hand. Several times she reached up and stroked my bald head.

"You're not going to die today," she said matter-of-factly.

I stared hard into her eyes and asked, "How do you know that?"

She just smiled and said, "You're not going to die for a long time. You have a lot of work to do. But the only thing you need to do today is rest."

She then became very animated, asking me about my children, telling me about hers. They were grown now, she said, but there was a lullaby she had sung for them when they were little that always helped them fall asleep. She asked if I would like to hear it, and I nodded.

Susan began to sing in the sweetest voice I have ever heard. The melody was simple and the words were about peace and healing and wholeness. It was an odd lullaby, but strangely comforting. It made me feel safe, and I fell asleep. I awoke off and on during the next several hours. Each time I opened my eyes, Susan was sitting right there, smiling at me, stroking my arm and singing her lullaby.

When I awoke late in the afternoon, she was gone. I felt energized and strong, as if I had just had the best night's sleep of my life. I was pulling myself up as the nurse who had started my IV came into the room.

"You look like you're feeling better," she said as she began to shut down the IV pump and disconnect the tubing from my catheter.

"I feel great," I told her. "A hundred percent better."

"Great!" she said. "Then let's get you up and out of here."

As she helped me get dressed, I told her I needed to see Susan before I left.

"I can't believe she stayed with me all day," I said. "I know she must have had other patients to tend to..." My voice trailed off as I saw the puzzled look on the nurse's face.

"There's no one here named Susan," she said. "I'm the only one who's been in and out of the room while you've been here."

I was the only one who had seen Susan. She had been there just for me.

If you're like most people, you are thinking that I fell asleep and dreamed her, that I was so ill I was delusional, or that I experienced a drug-induced hallucination of some kind. All three are very real possibilities, and it is even likely that at least one of them is true.

But the point I want to make here is that it doesn't matter! What matters is that Susan came to me in a way that I could understand in the darkest hour I have ever experienced. Her voice, her touch, her smiling eyes, her song and her words healed me at the core of my being. There is no doubt in my mind that Susan was an angel, but it took me many months to begin to see this and several years before I could accept it and talk about it openly.

My encounter with Susan and her conviction that I was not going to die that day undoubtedly gave me strength and courage to face the rest of my chemotherapy and the radiation treatments that followed.

But its lasting effect has been twofold. First, it opened my eyes and my spirit to receive the angels who surround me every day, who come to me in the guise of a tender gesture from my husband, a surprise visit from one of my sons, a butterfly resting for a moment on my shoulder, or just a bit of good news here and there. Second, it instilled in me the profound belief that, even in life's darkest hours – no, *especially* in life's darkest hours, when all seems lost and we feel utterly alone and abandoned, our angels are with us. No matter what the outcome of the experience, they are our unfailing companions, ever present to guide and advise, to comfort and console. We just have to be willing to be quiet so that we can hear their lullabies.

It doesn't matter how our angels reveal themselves to us. It only matters that they come when we need them. And they do. And they will. Without fail. Every time.

I believe I began to get well that day because I *believed* I was going to get well. Susan had said so.

My encounter with Susan helped me begin to heal in many ways. Understanding at some level (but not yet ready to admit openly) that the encounter had been a spiritual one, I began a conscious and consistent effort to open myself to the possibility of other spiritual events. I looked for meaning and messages in every meeting with every person, loved one or stranger. I tried to learn from every experience, routine or unusual.

This new approach was not easy because I had never lived my life this way. It required effort, and that effort became the focus of every day. It required frequent reminders to myself and repeated redirection when I found my mind wandering back to fear. But in hindsight, I realize it became easier each day because I *wanted* something else to focus on. This new and intriguing approach to life was a welcome relief from the fear I had lived with – not just since our cancer diagnoses, I now realized, but my whole life.

I had to force myself to ask the questions: What is this experience supposed to mean? What am I supposed to learn from this person? How can I grow from this pain? And finally, how can I use all of this – the sum of my life events – to heal myself and then somehow give back and share with others what I've learned?

The first steps in spiritual growth, I quickly learned, are like a baby's first steps when learning to walk. "Spiritual babies" take missteps and fall down a lot. But just as a baby doesn't stop trying to learn to walk because he falls down, we can't allow missteps and tumbles to halt our efforts.

One of my first attempts at spiritual awareness came in, of all places, the post office. For months, I had not had the strength or energy to run even the smallest of errands, and that loss of independence had been one of the most frustrating aspects of my illness. As I began to regain some of my strength and energy, it became very important to me to reclaim little tasks. I was still so weak, however, that if I needed to go to the post office, the dry cleaner and the grocery store, I was likely to have to come home and rest after each stop before heading to the next.

So on that day, I found myself standing in a very long line at the post office to buy stamps. Only one window was open, and the clerk who was manning it seemed to be moving in slow motion. The line had not advanced for what seemed like forever.

I was nauseated and weak in the knees. Just standing in that line required focused effort. I had to think hard and talk to myself, and I had to will myself not to sit down right there on the floor of the post office.

Two women ahead of me in line began to complain first to each other and then loudly to everyone within hearing distance. They clearly wanted the postal clerk to hear them, too. They made repeated comments like, "This is ridiculous!" and "I've been standing here for twenty minutes without moving!" and "What on earth is going on here? Why don't they open another window? Has everyone in this place gone to lunch?"

Then one of them said, "I've got better things to do than stand in this line all day!"

I thought about this and then wondered, *Do I have anything better to do today than stand in this line?*

And then the answer: *Nope.*

I continued the conversation with myself, trying to figure out what this experience meant. *After I stand in this line, I will go home and lie down. I will breathe in and I will breathe out and I will say "Thank you!" to God for letting me be alive one more day. I will say "Thank you!" for letting me stand in this line on my own two feet under my own power, for not letting me fall down, for allowing me to buy stamps all by myself without anyone having to help me or drive me to the post office or drive me home… Thank you! Thank you! Thank you!*

I call this experience my "grace moment." In that instant, in that dull, gray, slow-motion government building, I suddenly – and without warning! – found joy in *just being alive in that moment.* I literally felt elation saturate my whole being, like my soul had been flooded with adrenaline. It was exactly like falling in love and, in a way, I guess that's exactly what it was. I tingled all over, right to the tips of my fingers and toes. I was quite certain I was glowing.

In the very first seconds of this life-altering event, however, I thought I was having the mother of all hot flashes! But then my stomach stopped roiling. My knees stopped knocking. I smiled a little, and then I started to giggle as I realized what was happening.

I had discovered the power of gratitude from whence all true joy emanates.

In that same instant, I felt overwhelming compassion for the two complaining women. I actually felt sorry for them. They just didn't "get it." I said a silent prayer and asked for blessings on them.

For a split second, I actually considered saying to them and even shouting to everyone in line, "Do you know how lucky you are to be standing here? Do you have any clue how many people would gladly trade places with you just for the privilege of standing in this line? Don't you get it? You're alive in this moment! Be grateful!"

Thank goodness I realized before I opened my mouth that the post office is probably not the best place to initiate a confrontation, even a well-intentioned one. Can't you just see the expressions on people's faces had I said aloud what I was thinking? Can't you just see those nearest me stepping backward, trying to move away from the crazy lady?

And isn't it ironic that the two complaining women didn't get those kinds of looks or reactions, but my remarks certainly would have?

We have all become so accustomed to the negativity and joylessness in the world around us that we don't even notice them anymore, yet it makes everyone nervous when someone starts spouting off about joy and gratitude and being in the moment.

My days were becoming more bearable thanks to some of the "life lessons" cancer was teaching me. But the nights were still hard. In fact, the worst times by far were the nights.

I often awoke around two or three in the morning and couldn't go back to sleep. As I lay in bed listening to Roger's breathing, my imagination took hold and painted scary pictures. I imagined Roger's life without me which in turn led to picturing my sons' lives without me which led to yet more thoughts of all that I would miss: their high school graduations, their college and career choices, their weddings and babies. As the sadness washed over me, it was often replaced by terrifying images of my own funeral, visions of my body in a coffin, of my husband and parents and my precious boys weeping and inconsolable and me not there to comfort them. Not knowing how to *not* think about these things, I spent many tortured nights that I now know were unnecessary.

I was chatting one day with an elderly man sitting next to me in the communal treatment room at the oncology clinic. As our "chemo cocktails" dripped down our IV tubes into our bodies, I mentioned to him my bouts of terrified wakefulness in the wee hours. He responded that he had once had them, too.

"But now I call them 'God's Night Classes'," he said.

I was dumbfounded.

He continued. "Did you ever stop to think maybe the reason you wake up in the middle of the night is because God woke you up?"

"Why would God wake me up?" I asked suspiciously. "Just so I can lie there in the dark and be scared to death?"

"No," this very wise man replied. "Because it's quiet then, and you can have an uninterrupted conversation with Him. He's inviting you to talk to Him and, more importantly, to listen. The next time it happens, instead of lying there and allowing frightening imaginings to overtake you, think of yourself as safe, cradled in God's lap. Talk to Him. Tell Him where it hurts. Tell Him what you need. Then listen. And trust."

I never saw the man again. I asked the nurses about him from time to time, and they told me what a cheerful patient he was. Months later, I learned he had died.

What a blessing his brief presence in my life had been! His advice caused yet another shift in my perception of what was happening to me. He had handed me the bud of a realization that would take several years to blossom into awareness, the beginning of my understanding that our *interpretation* of any given situation or experience *is* its reality.

By this time, I had been selected by the computer to receive the trial drug Taxol. Even though it meant four more cycles of chemotherapy, I was so happy! It meant I had yet another weapon in my battle with cancer. While that drug does not, in most cases, cause the debilitating nausea patients can experience with some other cancer-fighting drugs, it can cause severe joint and bone pain as well as numbness in the hands and feet. I spent many days sitting on the couch with heating pads wrapped around both wrists and both ankles.

But my encounters with Susan and the old man at the clinic as well as my "post office epiphany" had calmed my spirit. I felt more hopeful every day. What I didn't realize then was that these spiritual experiences had literally rocked my world – and everything I had ever believed – on a seismic scale that even cancer couldn't rival. I had confronted the brick wall of my own mortality, accepted and then embraced it, and finally found my way to the other side.

I had my last chemotherapy treatment on my mother's birthday, August 23, 1996. I think it was the best birthday present I have ever given her.

While I was thrilled to be finished with the treatment drugs and their side effects, radiation still lay ahead. I knew nothing about radiation, and I knew no one else who had been through it. Although the transition from one type of treatment to another signaled that I was making progress and actually getting *through* all of this, it was yet another unknown in what had come to be a year of unknowns.

Ready or not, I was learning to take one leap of faith after another.

CHAPTER 5

Learning to Lighten Up

L
ike most cancer patients, I looked forward to my hair growing back once my chemotherapy treatments ended, but it would be quite a while before I felt comfortable going out in public without my wig. As I moved from chemotherapy to radiation treatments at the end of that long, hot summer, a funny thing happened. Literally!

One steamy afternoon, I'd had just about all I could take, and I was in a *very* bad mood. In spite of the fact that I was becoming more hopeful and less depressed thanks to the several enlightening experiences described earlier, I still had my bad days. This had been one of them. Sitting in my car at a red light, I was hot and tired and eager to get home to our air conditioned house.

I was also still stinging a bit from a conversation with Roger earlier that morning during which he had told me I needed to "lighten up a little."

"Where's your sense of humor?" he had asked me.

It irritated me that he found it so much easier to laugh than I did. I *wanted* to laugh, but just couldn't seem to find the humor in what we were all going through.

Noticing that my wig felt lopsided, I took advantage of the red light to look into the rear view mirror. I tugged on the sides and front of the wig to straighten it and saw, to my horror and embarrassment, four teenagers in the car behind me mocking my movements! They were modeling in exaggerated fashion the primping of a vain woman posing before a mirror, and they were laughing themselves silly.

My eyes filled instantly with tears of humiliation. *How could they be so cruel?* I wondered. *How could they make fun of a sick woman?*

Because they don't know, I quickly answered myself. *And besides, they're just kids. Come on, Kathy,* I imagined my husband saying. *Lighten up a little. They don't know any better.*

Then I thought b*ut they should.*

I don't know where it came from – maybe I was delirious from the heat – but a giggle bubbled up inside me and, without another thought, I placed my right hand on top of my head and yanked off my wig. Still looking in the mirror, I gave a huge shrug of my shoulders and laughed out loud just as the light turned green.

I will never forget the look of total shock on those four teenagers' faces as I pulled away from the intersection. All four had their hands to their cheeks, and their mouths and eyes were as big and round as dinner plates. I can still hear the horns of other cars blaring at them to move as they sat there stunned and motionless.

I didn't stop laughing for three days. And, for the most part, I haven't stopped laughing since. Because what I discovered that day was that the physical act of laughing made me feel *physically* better.

Now a lot of people – including Roger – had been telling me for a long time that "laughing will make you feel better," but I thought they meant on some higher, esoteric level, and my head and heart just hadn't been in the mood for that.

What I hadn't understood was that laughing would make me feel *physically* better. And that, in fact, laughing would make me *physically* healthier.

Once I *made* myself laugh by removing my wig to shock those young people, I realized I could make myself laugh pretty much any time I wanted to.

Compared to chemotherapy, the radiation treatments were a cake-walk. Like anything unfamiliar, the procedures and the huge pieces of equipment were overwhelming and scary at first, but I soon got used to them and settled down into the routine of driving to the hospital every day, undressing, climbing onto the table and lying still, dressing and driving home again. There wasn't much more to it than that.

The oddest thing (and, again, something no one had prepared me for) was having to be marked (temporary marks) and tattooed (permanent!) for the radiation treatments. At my initial appointment, the radiation oncologist examined me, took some measurements and made some notes. He then turned me over to the team of radiation technicians who would administer the treatments.

One of these technicians explained that she would be making some marks on my chest after doing some calculations. She would also be putting a small tattoo (she said it would "look like a dot from a ballpoint pen") between my breasts and another one under my arm. These marks and tattoos would guide the technicians as they readied me for each treatment so that the complicated calculations would not have to be done over and over.

As she prepared to tattoo me, I nervously joked that, as long as I had to get a tattoo, it was a shame it couldn't be something pretty like a rose or a heart. She just smiled.

When she was finished, she told me to sit up and gave me a hand mirror. There between my breasts was a beautiful pink rose tattoo! It was a rub-on tattoo, of course, but the significance of the gesture took my breath away. This technician in this cold, tile-and-steel treatment center had done something supremely human and kind for me. She had given me something pretty during a time when I felt hopelessly ugly.

The five weeks of radiation treatments were really little more than an inconvenience. I suffered no ill effects other than some mild dryness of the skin in the radiated area and a little more fatigue than usual. I was so glad to be finished with chemotherapy that I was able to ignore these minor symptoms for the most part. I guess everything really is relative.

My last treatment was the week of my own birthday. There was finally light at the end of this long, dark tunnel, and my spirits were beginning to lift a bit. I took a cassette tape of the theme from "Rocky" with me and played it as I drove home from the hospital for the last time.

Although my treatments were over, the medical tests and doctor's appointments were not (nor, I was beginning to realize, would they ever be). Dr. Mason explained my follow-up care. I would see him every three months for the next two years. If I was doing well at that point, the length of time between visits would become longer. After five years, I would still need to see him once a year for the rest of my life. He reminded me frequently that breast cancer can recur many years later; it is not one of the cancers patients can quit worrying about after five years.

I told Dr. Mason that I was really struggling with the fear of a recurrence and wondered what he thought of support groups for cancer survivors.

He was hesitant. "Some are better than others," he said. "As a rule, I don't recommend them. Patients tend to forget that every case is different and they begin to compare their treatments and outcomes to those of others in the group."

He told me that, if I decided to join a support group, it would be a good idea to visit several and to choose one that was professionally facilitated.

"Just because someone in the group may have had a recurrence of her cancer doesn't mean that you will," he continued. "You have to remember that your case is different from everyone else's. By all means, go to one or two meetings and decide for yourself. If they help you, fine. But if you find them upsetting, stop going. My guess is that now that your treatments are over, you will find yourself worrying less and less, and your life will start getting back to normal."

Oh, good Lord, not that! I thought. *At our house, "normal" is just a setting on the dryer!*

I visited several support groups for breast cancer survivors before settling on one held monthly at a nearby hospital. As Dr. Mason had predicted, there were women in various stages of disease and treatment. Some were extremely ill, and seeing them made me realize how far I had come in just a few short months. There is a special bond between women who have had a breast cancer experience, and I immediately liked the women in the group.

It was the facilitator who made the meetings unpleasant and unproductive. She was a very young nurse who had obviously been handed the assignment of leading the group. She was not a cancer survivor and, in fact, had no experience whatsoever in the oncology field. Worst of all, she had no idea what breast cancer survivors needed or wanted to talk about in a support group. She gave us a printed list of speakers who would be giving presentations at upcoming meetings on topics of absolutely no interest or value to us. She lectured us and recited canned advice. Occasionally she even made thoughtless comments about a group member's good test results ("I wouldn't put all my trust in that test. It's not very reliable.") or length of survival ("Congratulations on your two-year anniversary, Beth. Just remember your cancer can come back at any time."). We often had to comfort one another after a meeting because of something the facilitator had said.

At one meeting I attended, a young woman of about thirty sat next to me. She was a little plump and very attractive, and there was an air of mischievousness and fun about her. She introduced herself as Juanita.

As the facilitator dominated the meeting with her clichés, Juanita mumbled funny comments under her breath. When the nurse encouraged us to "tell your loved ones what you need," Juanita muttered, "What I *need* is to get out of here and away from her." I laughed, and the two of us began a whispered conversation.

We talked about the support group, how frightening it was to see the ones who were so sick, and how poorly equipped and trained the facilitator is. We learned we had been diagnosed at around the same time and briefly described our experiences to each other ("How many chemo treatments did you have to have?" "Did you have radiation?"). Then we decided to leave during the break and go to the hospital coffee shop.

Over sodas and pie, we discussed how we felt about the support group. While we cared deeply about the other women, we agreed that our foremost responsibility was to our own health and that, if the group only made us sad and angry, then it was not healthy for either of us.

We shared our stories with each other and talked about the fear. Juanita was shocked to hear about Roger's and my simultaneous diagnoses. I learned that Juanita had never been married and lived with her younger sister. Their mother was ill and, although they had a father and brothers, the family was not close.

Juanita's surgery had been much more extensive than mine. She had undergone a modified radical mastectomy and was considering reconstructive surgery.

She said, "The only thing I've ever really wanted is to have my own family. You know – a husband, kids, the house with the picket fence and a puppy in the yard, that whole thing. Having cancer has made me realize that time flies whether you're having fun or not. So I'm thinking I'd like to have the reconstruction done. If I feel better about the way I look, I think I'll find it easier to go out socially and meet people. It can't hurt, I guess. At the very least, I won't walk lopsided anymore."

We were paying our tabs and getting ready to leave while she was saying all of this. Her last comment puzzled me until she led the way out of the coffee shop. She walked in an exaggerated lopsided manner, looking a little like the quintessential assistant to the mad scientist. I laughed all the way to my car.

Juanita and I visited several other support groups together, but we never found one that made us feel "supported." One group we visited was for patients with all types of cancer. It was even worse than the first one we had attended. Every patient there was much older than either of us, and most were either in the very last stages of illness or the spouses of patients who had recently died. When we left, we were both in tears.

We had lengthy discussions about whether to try more support groups.

"No matter what group we go to, there are always going to be people sicker than we are," I said.

"True," said Juanita. "And if all that does is scare us and make us depressed, then we probably shouldn't go, right?"

"Maybe. But don't we have some kind of moral obligation to be there to support the people who are worse off than we are? Because some day we might be the ones who are worse off, and don't we want people to be there to support us?"

"True, but if going and seeing these people and watching them die makes us more depressed, and if depression and grief reduce your immune system's ability to fight disease, aren't we setting ourselves up for recurrences of our own cancers by repeatedly exposing ourselves to that kind of sadness?"

We went back and forth, finally making a decision that support groups just weren't for us. We did want to do something to "give back" and to help others with cancer, though, and we eventually became involved in an event called "Relay For Life" sponsored by the American Cancer Society. Relay For Life raises money for that organization's research, education and patient support services. It's basically an overnight, family-friendly community party, usually held at a local football stadium or venue big enough for hundreds or even thousands of people to camp out in overnight. Today there are more than 4,000 Relays For Life throughout the United States and the world. Roger, Juanita and I decided Relay was the healthiest "support group" for us.

Several weeks after meeting Juanita, she was hospitalized for the first of several procedures to reconstruct her breast. When I went to visit her, I found her sleeping.

She opened her eyes and said, "I lied."

"About what?" I asked.

"Remember when I was thinking about having this done and I said 'it can't hurt'? I lied. It hurts like hell."

"Yeah, but think how gorgeous you're going to look when you're all done. You'll have the perky breasts of a seventeen-year old!"

She laughed and winced. "Don't make me laugh, dammit! It hurts!"

Juanita and I had been good for each other in just the few weeks that had passed since we met, and Roger had also taken an instant liking to her. Because the three of us had been through much the same experience, our friendship deepened quickly. Each of us had a new respect for life, its unpredictability and brevity. We had all come to realize there is no point in moving slowly or taking your time to think about doing things that you know are right for you. If it's right and good, do it. This includes everything from surgery to improve one's self image to making new friends.

A nurse entered the room to check on Juanita. Juanita introduced me as her "breast friend."

My friendship with Juanita had helped me continue to "lighten up." She cracked me up every time we talked on the phone or got together. And while Roger's natural good humor had carried him a long way, Juanita's dry wit and sharp observations helped lift his spirits even higher. She was feisty and funny, and just being around her was good medicine for anyone.

The horrible year that had been 1996 finally came to an end. Roger and I had a new friend, renewed health and strength, and a new attitude. Life was very, very good indeed.

MARATHONS...

CHAPTER 6

The Darkest Hour...

We were all very different people from the ones we had been the year before. Roger was fully recovered from his surgery, and we were hopefully optimistic that his battle was over. His amazing sense of humor helped all of us over the rough spots. He was able to find something funny in virtually every situation, whether it was an overdue bill, an upcoming medical checkup or the car breaking down.

While my overall health and state of mind were improving, cancer treatment had taken its toll. Because my hair was growing back and I was beginning to look like myself again, everyone around me assumed I felt as healthy as I looked. Nothing could have been further from the truth. Certain side effects would linger for years and some perhaps forever, although I didn't know it at the time.

The worst of the lingering side effects was an inability to concentrate or focus, and sometimes to even think clearly. Always an avid reader, I started countless books, but never got past a chapter or two. Driving familiar streets in my hometown, I occasionally experienced waves of panic as I realized I didn't know where I was, where I was going or how to get home. When this happened, I just drove around and around until my thoughts cleared again. I never told anyone about these episodes for fear my family would have me admitted to a psychiatric hospital, and I'd had enough of hospitals and drugs and doctors of any kind.

The last year had turned our sons from giddy teenagers into quiet, often somber young men. Ryan found it so difficult to hear or talk about cancer that he simply left the room whenever the subject came up. Reid was willing to talk about it, but such conversations left him visibly shaken. We worried about them constantly, wondering what they were thinking and whether we had handled our cancer experience "the right way" in terms of helping our children cope with it. While we reminded ourselves there probably was no "right way" and acknowledged there had been no road maps that we knew of for helping children cope with the cancer diagnoses of two parents at the same time, we spent a lot of time thinking of things we believed we "should have" done.

Juanita had become a part of our family, and her frequent visits always brought a burst of sunshine into our home. She was raucous and sometimes bawdy. Her good humor was always infectious.

It seems now that all of us – Roger and I, Ryan and Reid, our parents and other family members as well as all of our friends – spent the next eighteen months just trying to regain our balance, to recover from the psychological and emotional onslaught of cancer. We realized that, for better or for worse, we would never be the same again. A certain amount of grieving comes with that realization, but there is also a sense of excitement about what the future holds and how the past will impact it. It is a very odd mix of sadness and elation.

Every day was bittersweet now. Old clichés that had once made me gag ("Today is the first day of the rest of your life!") now made sense. We had learned so much from our "cancer experience."

On most days, life completely overwhelmed us with its beauty and magic. Instead of cursing a sudden storm that ruined an outing, we eagerly waited for it to end so we could run outside and see and smell the freshly washed world. If we were really lucky, there would be a rainbow. Dark clouds and silver linings and all that. Yes, trite as it may seem to those who haven't been "there," every experience became a metaphor. Irritations that had once annoyed or even angered us seemed trivial. Even serious matters became less worrisome when we reminded ourselves that "Hey! At least it's not cancer!"

The telephone rang late one afternoon in June of 1998.

"I need you to go to the doctor with me," Juanita said.

"Sure," I said. "What's wrong?" There is was again, that old sensation of ice water in my veins.

"I don't know yet. Some of my counts were off when I had my blood work last week, so they called me to come in and have it done over. I did, and they just called me to come in tomorrow at 4:00 so Dr. Kelly can talk to me about the results. I don't want to go by myself."

"No problem," I said. "I'll pick you up at 3:30. But I'm sure it's going to be okay, Nita. He's just going to tell you the first results were wrong, and the second test showed that everything is fine." I knew I was lying.

She did, too.

"You know that's not true," she said. "If everything is fine, they either don't call you at all or they call you and say everything is fine. It's only when everything is *not* fine that they tell you to come in."

I continued to lie.

"Well, I'm sure if there is something wrong, it's something minor and they'll fix it."

I didn't even sound convincing to me.

"It'll be okay, Nita," I said. "I promise."

I replaced the receiver and told Roger what Juanita had said.

He took a deep breath and blew it out. Then he pulled me into his arms.

"You okay?" he asked.

"No."

"Me neither."

I picked Juanita up the next afternoon and drove her to the clinic. She didn't speak at all during the trip. When we sat down in the waiting room, she said, "I'll go in by myself. If it's bad, I'll send for you."

Juanita's name was called, and in less than five minutes, a nurse called my name. I rushed back to the small examining room where

Juanita sat huddled in a chair. She was pale and shaking, her eyes glazed over as if all the life had just drained out of her. I sat in the chair next to her and pulled her toward me in a protective hug.

"What? What is it?" I asked Dr. Kelly.

"Juanita's cancer has metastasized to a number of vital organs," he said. "I have explained to her that we cannot make her well. We can begin chemotherapy treatments and hope they will shrink the tumors or at least slow down their growth, but we cannot cure her."

A nurse came into the room with a sedative and a cup of water. Juanita swallowed the pill, but it was clear she was going into shock. She was almost unresponsive.

The doctor continued talking. He spoke of "quality of life issues" and "keeping you comfortable." I knew what he was saying and, if Juanita heard him at all, I was sure she understood, too.

He was saying she was going to die and probably fairly soon.

He left the room saying we were welcome to stay as long as we liked.

When he was gone, Juanita looked at me with the saddest eyes I have ever seen and slowly shook her head back and forth. I pulled her again into my arms like a mother would a child, and we sat like that for long minutes.

Words fail us at times like this, but now I know that maybe it's for the best. Sometimes our hearts are at their most eloquent when they compel our mouths to be silent. Juanita knew what my heart was saying. I loved her like a sister, and I would be there for her no matter what.

Within minutes, she said, "I need to get out of here."

In the months that followed, Juanita cycled over and over again from denial to depression. Sometimes she spent days in denial and so was cheerful and optimistic, insisting she would "live to be eighty." Other times she spent days in deep depression. And at other times, she cycled repeatedly over the course of minutes or hours, even within the same brief conversation.

She lost weight rapidly, whether from her disease or the treatments, I didn't know. I remember a day that summer when I thought she had never been more beautiful.

We had invited her to come over for a swim in our backyard pool. She had lost about twenty pounds and bought a new bathing suit to fit her newly slim body. The suit was a shiny, metallic green that flattered her fair skin and eyes.

As she stood on the deck, poised to dive into the pool, late afternoon sunlight reflected off her in such a way that the green fabric took on the appearance of fish scales. Her body and the suit merged so perfectly in that moment that she looked like she might be transformed into a mermaid in the next. Suddenly she lifted and turned her head to look at Roger and me. She smiled at us, and for a moment, there on the deck by the pool in our backyard, she *was* transformed. She was ethereal. She sparkled. Roger and I gasped simultaneously as she smiled and dove into the pool.

That moment has become a snapshot we carry in our hearts.

As summer turned into fall, and as fall gave way to winter, Juanita became increasingly frightened. The treatments didn't seem to be working, and the side effects were debilitating. On one occasion, she had an allergic reaction to one of the drugs during an infusion and stopped breathing. Quick action by skilled nurses brought the situation under control, but the crisis so terrified her that she began to talk about calling a halt to the treatments, an option Dr. Kelly had told her was open at all times. It was a decision she didn't want to make, however. Ending the treatments or continuing them seemed equally ominous.

She became desperate and grasped at straws, insisting at one point on introducing me to a man she had met who claimed he could read people's "auras." An aura, he said, is a pattern of light waves that surrounds each of us, but only a gifted few can read them. He told us that Juanita's aura indicated serious illness, but that she would recover. My aura, he said, indicated robust health. The fact of the matter was that he already knew both of our diagnoses when he told us these things. I thought his act was pretty hokey but, for a while at least, Juanita took great comfort in his words. My only interest where he was concerned was to make sure he didn't take advantage of her in any way, whether financially, sexually or otherwise.

In time, my friend realized that her desperation, struggle, anger and denial were only robbing her of strength and energy. She reached a state of acceptance and began to prepare herself for the inevitable.

Juanita started seeing a therapist on a regular schedule and listening to meditation and relaxation tapes almost constantly. She read both of Dr. Bernie Siegel's books (*Love, Medicine and Miracles* and *Peace, Love and Healing*) and listened to his guided imagery tapes.

Thanks to Dr. Siegel's works and the compassionate counseling of her wise and very nurturing therapist, Juanita became during the last months of her life a serene young woman who had found a genuine spiritual connection to the universe and to God (to whom she referred as "Spirit"). Whatever the connection was (and she didn't often speak of it), it brought her great comfort and peace.

One Thursday evening in late January of 1999, she called and said she was in the mood for Mexican food and margaritas! We met at a local restaurant. Juanita was radiant and happy. She picked at her food, but downed several potent margaritas. I followed her lead, and she chose that we laugh a lot and talk only of happy things. I will cherish the memory of that evening forever.

Several days later, I left on the first of two back-to-back trips to Chicago to attend to some family matters. I told Juanita I would call her often and that I would be home in plenty of time to take her to her next treatment scheduled for the second week in February.

As I relaxed in my hotel room in Chicago, the phone rang. Roger's voice was shaky and subdued on the other end of the line.

"It's Juanita," he said. "She's gone."

"That's not possible," I said, knowing at the same time that, of course, it was true. "I just talked to her three days ago!"

He said she had suddenly become so ill she could not stand. She was admitted to the hospital, and her condition deteriorated steadily over the next twenty-four hours. She then drifted into a sleep which quickly deepened into a coma. She did not regain consciousness and died peacefully.

I replaced the phone in its cradle and walked to the window, leaning my face onto the cool glass and looking up into the dazzling blue sky of that bitterly cold February day. It was as if some part of me believed I could find her if I just stared at the sky hard enough and long enough. I was consumed with grief and guilt that I hadn't been there for her at the end.

Instantly, she let me know it was okay and that, in fact, it was the way she had wanted it. She reminded me of the great evening we had shared over margaritas, and she told me she was at peace. I am as sure of these things as I was of my brother's comforting touch in the moments following his death.

"I hope you meet my brother," I told her. "You'll like him."

CHAPTER 7

...Is Just Before Dawn

B y the following day, the news of Juanita's death had begun to sink in. Of course a part of me had known she was going to die, but another part of me was swept up in her manic moments, convinced as she was during those times that she would live to be an old woman.

Instead, she had died at the very young age of 34. Once she had said to me that all she ever wanted was to be a wife and mother.

It was so unfair, and my sadness turned to anger as I wandered around Union Station in Washington, D.C., waiting for the train that would take me home to Virginia. In spite of the anger, I was also feeling a nervous, jittery sensation tinged with anticipation and excitement, like the piling up of storm clouds. I had the strangest, strongest sense that the storm my life had become in recent years was about to break and that something truly amazing was about to happen, something that would transform me like summer rain transforms the landscape, making everything it touches bright and clean.

As I paced around the station, I passed an information counter that contained little stacks of brochures and pamphlets. A cardboard display stand held some other leaflets, but the only word visible was the word "AIDS." I pulled a brochure from the stand and sat down to read it.

The front of the brochure contained a photo of a man running. Below the photo were the words "You may not think you can do this, but you can." Intrigued, I opened the brochure.

And in that moment, in that small paper folder, I found the means by which I would take back my life. All the sadness and sickness, all the lessons and encounters with angels that had gone before, and all the love and loss in my life had laid the groundwork for change, but what I held in my hands offered the catalyst.

The leaflet explained that a new class of drugs called protease inhibitors could prolong the lives of AIDS patients and, in many cases, appeared to force the virus into dormancy that might allow patients to live normal life spans. These drugs, however, were very expensive, and most AIDS patients could not afford them. It went on to explain that the Whitman-Walker Clinic in Washington, D.C. was sponsoring the "National AIDS Marathon Training Program." Participants who raised a minimum of $1,700 for the purchase of these drugs for the clinic's patients would receive a six-month marathon training program and entry into the Marine Corps Marathon.

My heart was pounding by the time I finished reading the brochure. When I look back on that day now, I realize my excitement had nothing to do with participating in an elite running event. Other than high school gym class, I had never run so far as to the end of my driveway! I was a middle-aged, overweight breast cancer patient (I still didn't think of myself as a "survivor"), perhaps the least likely of all people to even think about running a marathon.

And, to be perfectly honest, I didn't even know what a marathon was.

My excitement came from the wording of the brochure and the way those words spoke to me of hope and confidence and courage. It *said*, "You may not think you can do this, *but you can*." It also quoted the powerful words of Eleanor Roosevelt: "You gain strength, confidence and courage every time you stop to look fear in the face. You must do the thing you think you cannot do." I mean, come on! Who was I to question that kind of conviction? Whoever had designed that little paper leaflet believed in *me*, and that was a peg I knew I could hang my sneakers on, if just for a little while. Just until I could begin to believe in myself again.

On the train ride home, I stared into the darkness outside the window. I thought about Juanita and all that she had wanted out of life, all that had been denied her. I sent a silent message into the darkness, blessing her and wishing her peace and wholeness. I felt her presence around me. *I'm fine,* she seemed to say. *Go on! Run your little race* (Juanita always had a gift for understatement) *or whatever you want, but don't waste a single minute. Get going!*

When I stepped off the train, I ran headlong into Roger's arms. He expected, he told me later, to see me swollen-eyed and tearful. Instead, he was welcoming home a joyful, grinning woman who was babbling about the Marine Corps and an endurance race and an AIDS clinic. He told me later that he thought grief must have caused me to lose my mind.

When he finally realized I was serious about running the Marine Corps Marathon, he was dumbfounded, to put it mildly. He knew I had never even been remotely athletic, except for one delusional summer twenty years before when I tried to learn to play tennis because I loved Chris Evert's outfits.

As a former athlete, Roger knew exactly what a marathon was and what training for one involved. He told me I would be in *way* over my head. He told me that serious runners spend years training to run a marathon, not months. He said he knew of world-class runners who entered marathons only to drop out miles before the finish line, sidelined by injuries and dehydration. He reminded me that the brochure said the weekly training runs were in Washington, D.C., a good five-hour drive from home.

I had a comeback to each of his arguments. Of course I did not intend to run competitively, I told him. My only goals would be to raise the money and complete the marathon. I would train by myself. I didn't need to go to D.C. for the training runs.

"There," I said. "Have I answered all your questions?"

"All but one," he replied. "Why? Why do you want to put yourself through this after all you've been through?"

I had to think for a few minutes before answering him because I wasn't sure I could put it into words. "I want to do this *because* of all *we* have been through. I want to do it for my brother and so that, just maybe, somebody else won't have to die from AIDS. I want to do it for Juanita. I want to do it for you and for me and because I'm sick and tired of all the dying and the misery and the sickness and because I want to fight back. I want to do it to show everyone that we're here and we're alive *today*. I want to do it because I *can*. *While* I can. And for everyone who can't." I paused. "And because Eleanor Roosevelt said I'll be stronger and braver if I look fear in the face, and that I have to do the thing I think I can't do."

Roger realized he couldn't talk me out of it. He shook his head and said, "You've lost your mind. And I love you."

The next day, I called the National AIDS Marathon Training Program and requested their information and registration packet. The person I spoke with was a bit skeptical when I said I couldn't come to D.C. on the weekends and that I would train by myself if they just told me what to do and how to do it. She said she would have someone call me back.

Later that afternoon, one of the trainers called. I told him about my brother's death from AIDS, Juanita's death from cancer, and about Roger's and my own battles with cancer. I told him I was forty-seven years old, overweight and out of shape, but that I was excited about this challenge and committed to doing whatever it took.

He wasn't skeptical at all. He said, "We have dedicated coaches and trainers who want you to succeed. If you do everything we tell you to do, and if you don't give up, you will cross the finish line of the Marine Corps Marathon."

CHAPTER 8

Gutting It Out

One of cancer's cruelest realities is that, for a while at least, it becomes who you are.

On a given day, you're a mom, dad, son or daughter living your life and minding your own business. You go to work or school, spend time with friends and family, enjoy projects and leisure activities, and make plans for the future.

The next day you are a cancer patient.

Everything changes in the instant you hear the word "cancer." Gradually, you come to understand that nothing will ever be the same again.

You realize that, even if you are one of the lucky ones whose cancer goes into remission, this disease is something you are going to have to think about and deal with for the rest of your life. At frequent and regular intervals from now on, your body will be poked, prodded, scrutinized and monitored for changes. Whether you have another two years or twenty-two years, cancer will always be your shadowy companion.

You see yourself differently. Others see you differently. Cancer is usually the first thing you think about when you wake up in the morning and the first thing others think about when they see or talk to you.

Your schedule goes from being filled with work, soccer games, hair appointments and countless other normal activities to being filled with medical appointments, surgeries, chemotherapy treatments, radiation treatments, and medication rituals.

You read about cancer, talk about it, think about it and even dream about it. News stories about cancer that you wouldn't have noticed before now become the focus of your attention.

Simply stated, you and those closest to you become obsessed with cancer. It's a normal response and, to a certain degree, a healthy one. On the positive side, it means that you stay on top of your appointments, follow your treatment team's instructions, and study and learn everything you can about your disease and treatment plan.

But the obsession can become a decidedly unhealthy one when it lasts too long and sets up an unending cycle of despair and suffering. When you are unable to enjoy respites from treatment and periods of remission, something is very wrong.

To some degree, that's what had happened to me. While I had enjoyed a lengthy period of emotional recovery and growth for a year and a half, Juanita's death had threatened to knock me back down. Cancer and all its sadness could have easily taken over my life again and once more become an unhealthy obsession.

Had it not been for the marathon.

In short, had I not replaced an unhealthy obsession with a healthy one.

Some will argue there is no such thing as a "healthy obsession," that the two words are mutually exclusive. I disagree. What I did was healthy for two reasons. First, I made a *conscious decision* to focus on the training program as a *life-affirming project*. Second, I knew the obsession would be a temporary one because it had a finite goal in the marathon itself.

A few days after I called the number on the brochure I had picked up at Union Station, a package of materials arrived in the mail. I couldn't wait to complete the forms and return them with my registration fee.

Within just a few more days, another package came. I tore it open and removed a National AIDS Marathon Training Program t-shirt. I pulled it on right then and there and began poring over the rest of the materials in the thick envelope.

Included were a number of fundraising supplies (sample letters and donor forms, envelopes, ideas for raising the money), a book (*Marathon!* by Olympian Jeff Galloway), a complicated-looking training schedule, and lots of information about how to spend the next six months of my life getting ready to run a marathon.

I read the book first. I learned what a marathon is, and I learned its history. The following is loosely quoted from Jeff Galloway's *Marathon!*

"The aggressive and militaristic Persians landed on the Plain of Marathon about 25 miles from Athens (around 490 BC), determined to conquer and enslave the citizens. When intelligence reports reached Athens noting that Persia had more than five times as many soldiers as the Athenians, plans were made to evacuate and burn the city before the invaders came…The volunteer Athenian army assembled in the hills above the Plain of Marathon to do battle…They wisely decided to send a messenger to Sparta to ask for support with troops and supplies. Phidippides ran about 130 miles to Sparta in a day and a half…The Spartan leadership decided to come to the aid of the Athenians, but not for 10 days as they were in the middle of an important community ritual. Phidippides ran back to Marathon and reported to the leadership, which prepared for an immediate battle. Their strategy was so brilliant that the Persians were repelled and ran for their ships. Phidippides was then dispatched to Athens to tell of the victory before the city could be burned. He covered the approximately 25 miles and said one magic word to the Athenian leadership: "Nike!" (Victory!). Athens would live, but the wounded and exhausted messenger died.

"When events were being considered for inclusion in the first modern Olympic Games in Athens in 1896, a friend of one of the organizers suggested that the run of Phidippides be commemorated in a footrace from the Plain of Marathon to the Olympic Stadium. The marathon was born and has been run in every one of the modern Olympic Games. The distance of about 25 miles was increased in 1908 when the Olympics were held in London. Organizers had already measured the course when the Queen mentioned that she wanted to watch the start. It only took a mention by a queen to extend the marathon course, and the extended distance became standard. A tradition among marathoners when passing the original finish distance at 25 miles is to say "God save the Queen!" or something like that. But considering Phidippides' run for reinforcements, today's marathoners are getting off easy – we could be running the equivalent of a 260-mile round trip to Sparta!"

Thanks to the Queen, today's marathon is 26.2 miles long.

So that was what a marathon was about. Distance and endurance. Courage and heart. Determination and pride. "Nike" had nothing to do with shoes.

I began to understand that, for beginners like me, a marathon is not about speed. It is not even about running pretty. It is about staying the course and finishing. Any way you can. Upright. On all fours. Flat on your belly if you have to. It is all about making it across that line.

Training would begin the first of May. The schedule itself was the most intimidating piece of paper I had seen since the treatment nurse had handed me my chemotherapy timetable three years before. This one began with five days of alternate walking and running for thirty to forty-five minutes followed by a Saturday run referred to in the schedule as "three miles easy."

Easy? I had never even *walked* three miles!

The schedule added time and mileage for each of the next twenty-six weeks, with the weekend "long runs" increasing gradually to eight miles, then jumping to ten and twelve miles, then switching to time-based runs of varying lengths, until a training run of twenty-four to twenty-six miles three weeks before the marathon.

This kind of training was like nothing I'd ever heard of – much less been a part of – and was so far removed from my realm of experience that I began to wonder if Roger (and, by now, everyone else I knew) was right when they said it was a shame I had fought so hard to survive cancer only to lose my mind.

Over the next few months, I read Galloway's book from cover-to-cover at least four times and studied other books on running. I always wore the t-shirt when I trained, and sometimes I slept in it. I called the marathon trainers and coaches in D.C. several times a week for moral support and to ask countless questions.

It all started to feel pretty good. For the first time in three years, my life began to revolve around something other than cancer. I had allowed cancer to define who I was for far too long. Now I was determined that the marathon would redefine my life.

When I began my training, I could barely walk the length of our driveway and back. A few weeks into the program, that distance increased to a few blocks. I walked and jogged mostly (I called it "wogging," a little shuffle that was sort of a walk and kind of a jog). When I tried to run, I quickly became winded and went back to walking. I crossed off the days on the training schedule, just as I had crossed off the days on my chemotherapy calendar three years earlier.

Because traveling to D.C. for the weekly group training runs was out of the question, and because I didn't want to be far from home if I got sick or hurt, I did all of my training on a quarter-mile track at the middle school in our neighborhood.

And because I was so slow, each Saturday long run took most of the day.

Knowing I needed help, I was glad to hear about a "Women's Beginning Running Class" at a local fitness center and eagerly signed up. What an eye-opening experience that was! I realized within the first few minutes of the first class that I didn't even qualify as a beginner.

The coaches asked us to introduce ourselves and tell how many miles we ran on average each week. The other women in the class were already running between twelve and twenty miles a week. When it was my turn, I said I had never really run, but was walking and jogging about an hour each day and following a training schedule that would have me running a marathon in a few more months.

The other women and the coaches were silent. I could almost hear them thinking, *"Oh, that poor delusional woman."*

Two of the coaches glanced at one another, then back at me. One said, "I'm sorry to say, but that's a pretty unrealistic goal. Runners spend years training to run their first marathon."

I was embarrassed, but told myself they just didn't understand. They didn't know about the training program, they didn't know about my brother or Juanita, and they didn't know about Roger and me.

The next week I wore a new t-shirt to class. On the back it said, "If you think running a marathon is hard, try chemotherapy." Showing a little attitude boosted my confidence.

When the class went out on training runs, I was left far behind. Sometimes one of the coaches would double back to check on me, but most of the time I was out there on my own. The other women in the class weren't being unkind or unfair; they were just serious about improving their own times and forms and becoming better runners. Holding back to keep me company would have kept them from achieving their own goals.

I did wonder about the coaches, though. It seemed to me one of them should have been inclined to help a real beginner learn to run (since that's what the title of the class stated), but they seemed uninterested in anyone who wasn't already an accomplished athlete.

Although this class was discouraging at times, it provided me on a July evening with an exhilarating experience I will never forget.

As always, after a half-hour or so of classroom instruction and discussion, the group moved outside to begin a training run on the three-mile trail that wound and looped through the woods around the fitness center. And, as always, I found myself alone after the first few minutes.

On that particular evening, I was a little over halfway through the marathon-training schedule, but I wasn't running yet. I still became winded easily and held back largely (I now realize) out of fear. Never having challenged myself athletically and still not trusting the state of my health, I worried about having a heart attack or other medical crisis if I pushed myself too hard. The marathon was less than three months away, and I wasn't even close to where I should have been at that point in the training schedule.

The weather that day was especially steamy, and a storm was moving in from the southwest as the training run began. The woods around me were eerily quiet as the comfortable chatter of the runners ahead of me faded away. Soon, the only sounds I heard were the rumble of distant thunder and my own slow, dull footsteps.

In a matter of minutes, the trail grew darker and the thunder nearer. Counting the seconds between the thunder and flashes of lightning, I knew the storm would soon move directly overhead. I became very nervous, knowing this trail, thick with towering trees, was a dangerous place to be. I was far enough along the trail that the distance back was about the same as the distance ahead, so my best option was just to keep moving forward.

I wondered why one of the coaches didn't come back for me. It was dark. I was alone and scared, and now I was mad.

How could they leave me out here by myself?

Anger and fear can be great motivators.

Just maybe, I thought, *if I move a little faster, I can get back to the fitness center before I get killed by lightning.*

I walked faster, then eased into a slow jog.

Suddenly, lighting crackled in the trees above me and thunder exploded overhead. The hair on the back of my neck prickled and stood on end.

And I began to run.

The rain came down in sheets. In a matter of seconds, I was soaked to the skin.

I had to take my glasses off because of the rain.

Now I was running blind.

The most dangerous part of the storm moved past quickly, but the rain continued to pound me. As I realized the threat of being killed by lightning was probably over, I relaxed a little.

No point in hurrying now, I thought. *I'm already soaked. Might as well enjoy the run.*

Enjoy the run. I'd heard others say it, but never knew what it meant.

The run.

That's when it hit me. I was running. Oh, my God, I was running! The feeling was totally foreign and completely wonderful.

For the first time, I heard the pounding of my own heart without being afraid of it. It sounded strong and healthy. I heard my breathing, and it was deep and powerful.

For the first time in my life, my body was in tune with the universe. My breaths were in sync with the wind in the trees. The rhythm of my footsteps and my pulse matched the beat of everything around me. I was hearing the hum and harmony of my own life; I was running to my own drummer.

It had only taken forty-seven years and a battle with the beast called cancer.

I relaxed into what I finally understood was an "easy" run. Not holding back, but not pushing too hard.

I still couldn't see because of the rain, but I didn't care. I even missed a turn-off on the trail causing me to run the same loop twice. I didn't care about that either.

I didn't care about anything except that I had really run for at least a mile, and *I hadn't thought about cancer the whole time!*

By the time I reached the end of the trail, the cars of the coaches and my running classmates were gone. It was okay. I didn't need them.

I leaned on my car and laughed and cried at the same time. I bathed in the warm summer rain as I swore never to forget how good this felt, how strong I was in this moment, how well I had taken care of myself and that, most of all – even if just for a little while – I had stopped being afraid.

The response to my letters to family members and friends requesting donations was overwhelming, and my parents threw a huge fundraising dinner party. I had even signed up with another marathon training program (the Leukemia/Lymphoma Society's Team-in-Training Program) because there were locally sponsored weekend long runs, and my family's efforts resulted in raising much more than the minimum required by both programs. With the fundraising requirements met, a certain amount of pressure was relieved, and I was able to give my full attention to running.

About this time, I received two very special gifts. The men at the Marine Corps recruiting office where our older son Ryan had recently enlisted gave me a red and gold (the Marine Corps colors) baseball-style cap embroidered "USMC Mom," and a friend of mine who worked at the Parris Island Marine Corps Recruiting Station in South Carolina sent me a cassette tape of Women Marines' running cadences. The hat became a part of my training "uniform," and the cassette tape became my daily inspiration and motivation.

I also ran a half dozen 5K races during the summer and early fall. I finished next-to-last or dead last every time, but I finished upright, without injury and without throwing up (which, due to coastal Virginia's brutal summer heat and humidity, was more than some could say!).

While my confidence level was higher than when I started, and while I no longer had the pressure of fundraising, I began to have serious doubts about being able to finish the marathon. I knew now what a marathon was, how hard it was just to finish a three-mile run, and how long it took my body to train enough to shave even a few seconds off my time.

I understood now that commitment is admirable, but the body needs more than commitment.

The great motivational speaker Napoleon Hill said, "Nature cannot be tricked or cheated. She will give up to you the object of your struggles only after you have paid her price."

I understood now that the body requires *training time*, and I began to believe that everyone who had told me six months wasn't nearly enough time had been right.

The trainers and coaches in D.C. now called often to check on me, and I discussed my concerns with them. I still walked and jogged more than I ran, I told them, and my time was nowhere good enough to finish in the allotted six hours. To complete the marathon in six hours, runners have to be able to maintain a 14-minute mile. My *best* mile was just under 14 minutes, so maintaining that for 26.2 miles was pretty nearly impossible.

And while most marathons are "walker friendly," the Marine Corps Marathon is not. The course is literally torn down after six hours, and (for insurance reasons) the race officials require "stragglers" to get on a bus. With the big day just two months away, I was still at a pace (if you could even call it that) that would take me much longer than six hours to finish. More than anything, I did not want to get on that stragglers' bus.

The marathon training staff assured me that coaches, trainers, and other personnel from the National AIDS Marathon Training Program would be on the course, stationed all along the miles; they would make sure all of the program's participants found their way to the finish line as long as they didn't give up.

"Just don't quit," one of the coaches told me. "No matter what the race officials tell you, you do not have to get on the stragglers' bus. Tell them your trainers will find you and be responsible for you."

"Okay," I said. "I can do that."

"Kathy," the coach continued, "whatever you do, don't quit. We will find you, and we will bring you in. If you don't give up, you will finish this marathon."

He also told me I would not be alone in terms of other runners. There were many participants, he assured me, who were not athletes, but who – like me – were doing this for personal reasons. He said I would meet them on the course because runners of the same pace eventually end up together.

With the marathon just six weeks away, I went out one morning for my training run. Everything was off that day. I was sluggish. My calves and feet felt full of lead. The soles of my feet burned, and I couldn't find my pace. Nothing was right.

The sports watch I had bought to calculate my splits (separate times for each mile) showed me my times were even worse than usual. It was the most disheartened I had been since starting the program. I was angry and discouraged when I came into the house.

Roger made the innocent mistake of asking, "How was your run?"

Before I knew it, I was ranting like a maniac.

"You were right!" I shouted. "I never should have started this stupid program! I'm making a fool of myself, and everybody has been able to see that except me!"

"What are you afraid of?" he asked.

I hesitated because I didn't want to admit it to him. But I finally blurted out, "I'm afraid I won't finish."

He waited for me to calm down. Then he said, "I am so proud of you."

Puzzled, I looked at him and said, "Why? I'm *horrible* at running! It is entirely possible I'm the worst runner there ever was!"

He asked, "Was that why you took this on? To become a runner? I thought you were doing this for your brother and for Juanita."

His simple reminder was the splash of cold water I needed.

In that instant, I knew I would finish the marathon, and I knew how I would do it. To this day, I don't know where it came from, but a plan began to take shape in my mind, a plan I would come to think of as my "secret weapon."

"I'll name the miles," I said. "I will name every one of those twenty-six miles for a person. I'll name one for you and one for me and one for each of our doctors and nurses, one for Ryan and one for Reid, one for each of our parents. I'll name one for everyone we know who has had cancer or AIDS. I'll finish the marathon because I could never live with myself if I quit during somebody's mile."

The plan continued to develop as I talked it out. Mile twenty-five would be mine.

And mile twenty-six would be my brother's.

I received two more amazing gifts that day, reinforcing my belief that God and the universe provide us with everything we need when we are moving in the right direction and being true to our reasons for being.

First, Roger said he would help me train. He had been an outstanding athlete in college and – while he didn't enjoy running, had never run a marathon and had no desire to do so – he felt he could draw on his experience to help me improve my times. At the very least, he said, he could offer me moral support and company. As he was still working ten-to-twelve-hour days to pay off the medical bills that appeared to have no end, he had precious few leisure hours. The time commitment alone was a huge sacrifice. I was moved and deeply grateful.

The second gift arrived by mail. It was my running singlet with the National AIDS Marathon Training Program logo on it.

It was official. Ready or not, I was going to run the Marine Corps Marathon.

CHAPTER 9

The Miracle of the Marathon

Sunday, October 24, 1999, was a cool, windy day with crystal clear blue skies over Washington, D.C. Roger and I walked from our hotel to the start of the race, which was about a half-mile away.

As we came over a hill, the sight that greeted us took my breath away. The sun was coming up over the spectacular Iwo Jima monument. There were 18,000 runners and close to 100,000 spectators gathered for the start of the race. A sea of people!

Roger and I made our way to the very back of the thousands of runners. I knew I would be so slow that I took my place far *behind* the last of the starting positions for the slowest runners.

We would hear many miraculous stories before that day ended. We would hear about a man who pushed his disabled son in a wheelchair the entire distance and finished long after midnight. We would hear about a woman celebrating her 83rd birthday who would need the assistance of others but who would go the distance and cross the finish line on her own two feet. We heard later that a couple actually got married at the start line. From my place at the "back of the pack," I could see the backs of hundreds of jerseys with names printed beneath them: "For Amy," "For my mom," "For Rick," "For children with AIDS." You just knew that every jersey with a dedication on it had a unique and powerful story.

The back of the pack had its stories, too. A woman near me was wearing a t-shirt that said "Wife of a cancer survivor." We had to talk to her, of course, and as we waited for the start of the race, we told her we were cancer survivors, too. She motioned us over to the side of the road where her husband was sitting in the shade of a tree. He was so weak and frail, but when she told him we were cancer survivors and that I was going to run the marathon, he stood up on shaking legs and hugged us.

He said to me, "Seeing you do this makes me believe I will be well and strong again some day."

I added one more person to the list I would carry with me on this day.

Roger kissed me, wished me luck and said he was going up front to see the start of the race. He would meet me at the finish line.

"You *will* finish!" he told me. "And I will be there to see you get that medal!" He hugged me again, told me how proud he was of me and disappeared into the crowd.

I pinned my race number to the front of my singlet. On the back of the singlet we had written "For my brother" with a felt-tipped marker. I began to stretch and to jog nervously in place. I was ready to do this.

The starting gun sounded in the distance. I was so far back that it took me 15 minutes to cross the official starting line! But I didn't care. There were hundreds of others back there with me, and hundreds more far behind us. A few of us shuffled along together, introducing ourselves and talking about the personal reasons we had taken on this challenge.

Only a few tenths of a mile in, we were overtaken by a small group of Special Olympians and their coaches. The group was made up of six young runners around the ages of eleven to fourteen. Their coach explained to us that these young people had Down's Syndrome and that they were in training for an upcoming Special Olympics event. He and his athletes had a goal that day of completing the first mile of the Marine Corps Marathon. It would be good training as well as a fun and exciting activity.

Around the middle of that first mile, one of the young athletes stopped and stooped down on the pavement. His shoelace had come untied. He slowly and deliberately began to retie the lace, but he was having some difficulty with it.

His companions missed him immediately, stopped, turned around and walked back to where he was now sitting on the ground, still struggling to tie that lace. At first, they stood over him and gave him verbal encouragement. Then they all sat down in a semi-circle in front of him and coached him on tying his lace. Finally, another youngster reached over and helped him tie it.

Then, grinning broadly, they all "high-fived" each other, stood, joined hands and took off running together. They disappeared quickly into the crowd ahead of us.

Yes, I had slowed down and even stopped to watch this most amazing scene. In my own heart, I knew that my only goal that day was just to finish the marathon. I had associated words like "winners" and "champions" with those people who I knew would finish the race in a couple of hours.

But in the minutes I watched those young Special Olympians, my definition of a champion changed forever. To this day, I don't know who won the 1999 Marine Corps Marathon, and I wouldn't know him if I saw him, but I can sure tell you who the champions were. I'd know them anywhere.

I began to think of this marathon as an unfolding of small miracles.

The first few miles went by quickly. The course was lined by spectators cheering all of us on. Each mile was marked by a large red number on a banner with Marines stationed nearby. These mile stations also had tables with cups of water and plastic bins of orange slices and bagel pieces.

As we passed the third mile marker, Roger was suddenly in step beside me.

I was stunned. "*What* are you doing?!"

"Well, I found out that the race officials will let anybody run, as long as all the registered runners have crossed the starting line. They call it 'bootlegging.'"

He shrugged. "I'm just going to go a few miles. I'll double back at six or seven and meet you at the finish."

Having him beside me was icing on the cake. I was thrilled to have my training partner, my best friend, my soul mate with me, even if it was just for a little while.

He told me about a woman he had met at the first mile marker. She had come to a complete stop and walked toward the side of the road. He asked her is she was okay, and she pulled off the scarf that covered her bald head. She said, "I'm in treatment for cancer right now. I just wanted to do the first mile."

One more amazing story. One more champion. One more miracle.

As the miles fell away, the runners spread out.

I asked Roger several times when he was going to double back, and he kept saying, "In a little while. I'll just go a little further with you."

A few times, I caught him looking a little worried. We passed mile markers 10 and 11 which took us by the Lincoln Memorial and the Washington Monument. He kept saying he would just go "a little further."

We passed mile marker 12 near the U.S. Capitol, went by Union Station, and then passed mile marker 13 on the far side of the Capitol. I didn't want to say anything, but I was starting to feel an added excitement.

I wasn't sure Roger even knew what he was doing yet, but I did.

Finally he said it. "You know, we're halfway to the finish line. Same distance either way. Guess I might as well keep going."

I literally jumped for joy. I threw my arms around his neck and kissed him all over his face. It had already seemed like a perfect day, but now I was even more certain that it was.

Occasionally a group of Marines noticed my "USMC Mom" hat and shouted, "Go, Mom!" We grinned and waved, damned proud to be Americans and parents of a United States Marine. Damned proud to be cancer survivors participating in an athletic event no one – including us – would have believed four years earlier that we could have entered, much less completed.

But we weren't there yet.

The landscape of the middle miles is lost in hazy memory now. I recall that the first 15 miles or so were fairly easy for us both. The training had paid off. The water and fruit stations were still up (although not at every mile marker now), so staying hydrated was easy, and energy was readily available.

As we neared the 17-mile marker, we could see Marines tearing down the banner. Other Marines were sweeping up the litter of water cups, and still others were breaking down the tables and other equipment.

One of the young Marines said, "Sorry, folks. The race is over."

Roger smiled at him and said, "Thanks, but we'll just keep on going if you don't mind." The Marine shrugged, handed each of us a large bottle of water and wished us luck.

That's when I panicked. "They're tearing down the course! It's been six hours and we've still got six miles to go, and now we won't even know where the course is! We'll get lost!"

Roger said, "Come on. Calm down. You knew this would happen. We won't get lost. Your coach told you they'd take care of you. They'll show up soon. Settle down and focus."

I did. I reminded myself of the people for whom I had named each mile. My secret weapon actually worked. I knew I wouldn't quit as long as someone showed me the way.

We entered a three-mile loop known as "Hains Point." Since we knew from the racecourse map that it was a loop, we knew that at least we couldn't get lost here.

Three other women had joined Roger and me around the time the course was torn down. One of them had a sprained ankle. She limped along as the other four of us shuffled along.

Suddenly, a white school-type bus pulled up alongside us. The stragglers' bus. A civilian driver leaned out the window and said, "Race is over, folks. You'll have to get on the bus now."

The woman with the sprained ankle was relieved to climb aboard, but the rest of us waved him on, indicating we had no intention of getting on the bus.

He drove slowly next to us and continued talking. "I'm afraid you'll have to. The course has been torn down and we can't be responsible for you anymore."

Roger said, "That's O.K. You go on. We'll be responsible for ourselves."

The driver shook his head, muttered "Damn fools" and drove away.

Without our injured companion, the four of us began to jog again. The two women with us introduced themselves as Lila and Kristin. They were also National AIDS Marathon Training participants.

This is where the training really began to pay off. This is where we learned what it meant to endure in an athletic event. We were exhausted, but we didn't care. We were sunburned (our sunscreen had long since been washed away by sweat) and in pain pretty much everywhere on our bodies, but we didn't care. All that mattered now was getting out of this loop and figuring out where to go next.

The day before the marathon, I had treated myself to a new pair of runner's socks for the occasion. That little indulgence had turned out to be a huge mistake. I literally had blisters on my feet that had formed on top of other blisters. Roger and I both had blood coming through the toes of our shoes.

Soon another bus pulled alongside. This one was a Marine Corps bus. It stopped, and a Marine Corps staff sergeant got off the bus. We kept hobbling along, and he fell in ahead of us, walking backward.

"You know you have to get on the bus now," he said. "This race is over. The course isn't even marked anymore. Once you get out of this loop, you won't know where to go."

We moved forward in silence because we didn't have energy to waste on words.

He grinned and spread his hands wide, talking to us like we were uncooperative children. "Come on. Get on the bus."

I'm not sure what made me do what I did next. Maybe it was a year of watching my brother die from AIDS. Maybe it was nearly four years of fighting cancer and watching it destroy Juanita's life. Maybe it was the marathon training program, and maybe it was everything in my life that had led up to this moment.

All I knew was that I was not afraid of anything or anybody anymore, not even a Marine staff sergeant. I honestly felt like I could hold my own with the entire Corps that day, if not on a physical level, then certainly on a mental one.

I kept moving forward, in step with him, and leaned in close. I was shaking as I spoke, not with fear but with determination. "You hear me, sir," I said. "This race is not over because we are not finished. We're not getting on your bus or the next bus or any other bus. Please leave us alone now."

He narrowed his eyes and glared at me. Then he simply nodded and said, "Yes, Ma'am." He got back on the bus, and it pulled away.

Today I like to pretend that he held some measure of admiration for us, but in reality I believe he thought we were idiots.

Kristin said, "You know, he's right. After we come out of this loop, we won't know where to go. I don't know where the finish line is, do you?"

The rest of us admitted we did not, but we reminded ourselves that the coaches and trainers had said they'd take care of us, that they'd find us and take us to the finish line.

Lila said, "Yeah, they did say that, but I don't think they really figured on anybody taking *this* long to finish. I'll bet they've all packed it in by now. Who could blame them?"

Finally, we could see the place where we had entered Hains Point. We had completed the loop. We had figured that, if anyone was going to meet us, this was where they would be.

But there was no one there. The area was deserted.

We kept moving silently forward, closer and closer to the spot from which we would not know where to go next, the place at which the marathon would be over for us, miles shy of the finish line.

Lila said, "Oh, my God. There's nobody there."

We stared at the spot in disbelief. I've never felt such bitter disappointment in my life. We had come so far, and now it seemed we would not be allowed to finish.

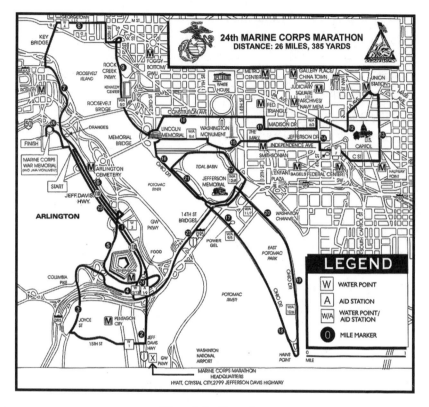

Map of the Marathon

Suddenly, from around a bend up ahead, a man appeared. He was wearing a National AIDS Marathon Training Program singlet, and he was holding a pole with a placard on it. The placard bore the logo of the program and the words "You are heroes!" He waved to us. The program had been true to its word.

Excitement and relief brought renewed energy. We whooped it up, cheered and shouted and high-fived each other as we ran to our rescuer. He told us his name was Dennis.

Practically falling all over each other and Dennis, and with all of us talking at once, we told him how worried we had been that no one would come for us, that we feared we were the last people on the course and that we were hopelessly lost. Worst of all, we told him, we thought it was over and that we would not be able to finish what we had come to think of as *our* marathon.

He said, "Didn't we promise you we'd take care of you?"

He told us our marathon was *not* over. We had six more miles to go.

Six more miles before we could claim our own miracle.

CHAPTER 10

My Brother's Mile

Dennis fell in with us and engaged us in motivational chatter for the next mile and a half which took us around the Tidal Basin. At the point where the mile marker for Mile 22 would have been, he handed us off to Anna, another program staffer. Anna would take us the next two miles, across the 14th Street Bridge to mile 24. Someone else would meet us there, she explained, and take us to the finish line.

As we neared the 14th Street Bridge, our little group spread out. Looking back, I think we began to realize at that point that we really were going to do this, we really were going to go all the way. Each of us needed a little room and a little quiet time for introspection.

The cold wind off the water whipped around me and shoved at my chest as if trying to push me backward. I leaned into it and pushed back. My face and lips were covered with salt from the sweat that had poured off me all day. Now the combination of salt and wind cut me, and I tasted blood.

The only reason I was moving forward now was that I had forgotten how to stop.

I was in what real runners and other athletes call a "zone." Zombie-like. Nothing could touch me. My body had long since stopped hurting. I had gone so far past pain that I didn't feel anything anymore.

My legs and feet were numb, but they continued to shuffle in the right direction, so I just trusted them to keep going.

Looking out over the Potomac River, I reflected on what this experience meant to me in this moment and what I believed it would come to mean to me in the years ahead.

On the simplest and most symbolic level, completing the marathon would mean that I had covered twenty-six-point-two miles in honor and celebration of twenty-six courageous individuals.

On another level, it already meant that I had learned what it means to live in the moment. I was here, right now, reveling in this achievement, alive and strong, my body doing amazing things I would not have believed possible four years earlier. I thought about every step I took. Each one was precious, and I savored it.

And on yet another level, I realized this day would become for me one of those cherished golden days that people relive again and again in their later years. We don't get very many perfect days in this life – maybe a handful or two if we're lucky. I knew this was one of mine. I wanted to remember how the salt tasted on my skin, how the wind felt when it slapped my face, what it all smelled and sounded like and the sights I had seen along the way. I thought about that long-ago day in the post office and reminded myself that all we really have to do is breathe in, breathe out and say "thank you."

I looked skyward and whispered a grateful prayer.

We came off the bridge and covered nearly another mile in silence. We had moved close to one another again, and some of us tried to speak to the others but couldn't. I don't know if it was total exhaustion or if we were in a mild state of shock, but the members of our little group looked stunned and shaky. We managed to murmur things like, "You okay?" and nod to each other, but nothing more. I noted that Anna often jogged backwards so that she was facing us. She was keeping a careful eye on our conditions.

We entered a small park where we were met by a program coach named Sean. After making introductions, Anna left us.

"How's everybody doing?" Sean asked.

No one answered. We just stared at him and nodded.

"I'm going to take you in now. Are you ready?"

Take us in? What did he mean? Take us in where?

I was confused, and the others in our group looked confused, too.

"Where are you taking us?" I managed to ask.

"To the finish line!" he said. "This is it, guys. You're at Mile 24."

It took a few heartbeats to sink in.

"This is it?" I asked, just to be sure.

"Yep," said Sean. "Let's go!"

"This is it." I had to say it out loud to convince myself.

Then I had to say it again. "This is it."

And again. "This is it!"

And then, "Oh, my God! This is it!"

I turned to Roger and shouted, "This is it! We're really going to do this! This is my mile!"

He grinned and said, "You go, girl."

And I went. We all went.

We were laughing and crying and high-fiving each other. We fell in beside Sean and just went for it.

I celebrated my mile by thanking God with each step for the miraculous and incredibly precious gift of a second chance at life. I had worked so hard for so long for this mile. Part of me wanted it to last forever. I counted every breath, every step, every heartbeat and filed them away in a secret place where I could keep them all my life. To this day, I often take them out and live them again.

Sean announced that we were at Mile 25. No one but Roger and I knew the significance of this moment to me.

I looked at Roger and managed to whisper, "This is my brother's mile. This one is sacred."

As I willed my trembling legs to carry me one more mile, I was overcome with emotion and grieved the tragic way my brother's life had ended. But I celebrated him, too. I celebrated his presence in my life for 34 years, his humor, his brilliance, his huge heart, his amazing blue eyes. I thanked God over and over again for the gift of a brother who had loved me.

I don't know at what point I realized that our bedraggled little group was running, perhaps not the graceful run of athletes, but the hell-bent, lopsided, limping run of wounded warriors and gleeful children. Suddenly, we were yelling and shouting for joy, whooping it up and making an incredible amount of noise. I wonder to this day where we found the energy.

As we neared the finish, more staffers from the National AIDS Marathon Training Program appeared along the way to cheer us on. Some were holding up the training program's "You are heroes!" placards.

As the beautiful Iwo Jima Monument came into sight, Roger and I joined hands. Lila and Kristin joined hands. We were ready.

But the finish line was nowhere in sight, and Sean had disappeared.

"Where is the finish line?" we asked the few people who were still along the road.

They applauded us, laughed and said, "Just a little farther. Keep going!"

We kept going. And going. And going. We began to think someone was playing a bad joke. We were right in front of the Iwo Jima monument which we knew to be the finish line, but we saw no "Finish" sign anywhere.

What we didn't realize was that the last few hundred yards of the marathon force the participants to go all the way *around* the monument. Those 385 yards are the longest of the course!

Finally, we saw it. Ours was not the big "Finish" sign we had seen in the brochures. Ours did not have the big digital clock over it to show us our times. Those things had been taken down hours earlier.

Ours did not have officials running to greet us with space blankets and sports drinks. Those people were long gone.

Our finish line was just a simple string lying in the grass, but it was the Holy Grail to us.

We ran full out now. I was determined to finish at a dead run.

As we neared the end, I felt a gentle tug on my arm. Roger was lagging behind me a few steps, but still gripping my hand. Wondering why he would hold back now, I glanced over my shoulder at him.

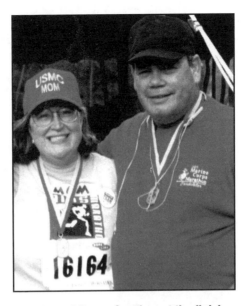

**Kathy and Roger Cawthon at the finish
line of the Marine Corps Marathon.
What a moment!**

He smiled and said, "You first."

Roger and I crossed the finish line together even though he let me take a step ahead of him.

Our time: 8 hours, 2 minutes, give or take a few.

But who cared? We had completed the Marine Corps Marathon. Officially or unofficially, it didn't matter to us. We were the only witnesses we needed.

It was several minutes before we calmed down enough to realize there were others around us. There were Marines. Lots of them!

And suddenly the Marine Corps Commandant was standing in front of us, his arm draped with beautiful, heavy medals on wide grosgrain ribbons in Marine Corps red and gold.

I removed my "USMC Mom" cap. The Commandant placed a finisher's medal around my neck, shook my hand and said, "Congratulations!" I thought I might die from sheer joy.

Then he did the same to Lila and Kristin.

But not to Roger. It was then I remembered Roger was a "bootlegger." He didn't have a race number because he wasn't a registered runner. With practically no training or support, he had accomplished an amazing feat. He had completed the grueling, 26.2-mile Marine Corps Marathon, and now he would have nothing to show for it.

He saw the look on my face and waved his hand in the air as if to say, "It's not important. Don't worry about it."

I could not accept that. Not now.

Pointing to him, I said to the Commandant, "He did it, too! The whole thing! He went the whole way!"

The Commandant said, "That's good enough for me." He placed a finisher's medal around Roger's neck and gave him hearty congratulations.

There was one more thing I had to do to make this a perfect day. I reached into the pocket of my shorts and pulled out a folded piece of paper, stained and wet with perspiration, ragged from being folded and unfolded too many times. It was my chemotherapy schedule, the one the nurse had given me on that awful day four years earlier, the one with more than fifty medical appointments on it.

The notations were still legible in all the little calendar squares: three surgeries, eight chemotherapy treatments, eight mid-cycle check-ups, two chest x-rays, a bone scan, a cardiac sonogram, an abdominal CT scan, a pre-radiation work-up, twenty-five radiation treatments and six radiation follow-ups. Each little square was marked through with a red "X." How I had hated that calendar, but because each crossed-out square meant one day closer to the end of my treatment, I had clung to it like a child to his security blanket.

Now it was time to let it go.

Roger looked over my shoulder and saw what I was holding in my shaking hands. He told those who were standing around us what it was.

Slowly and solemnly, I tore the paper into tiny pieces and tossed them into the air. Roger lifted me off the ground and swung me around. Marines, trainers and coaches applauded and shook my hand. The Commandant hugged and congratulated me again.

Damned if the only thing missing wasn't background music!

I have no idea who won the marathon that day, who placed or who set a record. I only know that, whoever those people were, their finishes could not have been more meaningful to them than ours was to us. In that moment, we had taken back what cancer and AIDS had stolen from us.

Twenty-six-point-two miles were nothing. Our journey had taken us so much further than that and had taught us so many priceless lessons along the way.

From my brother and from Juanita, we learned that, while every fight is not winnable, every warrior can persevere and each of us can write his own definition of "victory."

From our own battles with cancer, we learned that sometimes success means just showing up one more time.

And from the marathon we learned to never, ever get on the stragglers' bus. Finish or go down fighting, but don't ever give up.

I think Eleanor would have been proud.

...and MIRACLES

CHAPTER 11

Your Life Is a Miracle

This book is not about running marathons. We are not getting ready to encourage you to run a marathon (unless that's something you want to do), and we are not suggesting that running a marathon cures cancer or puts it into remission.

Up to this point, we have only told you what happened to us (simultaneous cancer diagnoses) and what we did afterward (we ran a marathon). Now we're going to tell you *why* we've told you those things and how you can use what we learned from all of that to create a better life for yourself after a cancer diagnosis. Our hope is that, by considering our story and its meaning and implications, you can skip much of the awfulness of that time between the diagnosis and deciding what *you* are going to do afterward.

First, you must know – *really know and accept and embrace* – that your life is a miracle! From the moment of your conception – which was a miracle in and of itself – miracles have occurred in your life and in your body every minute of every single day. Every function of your body, voluntary and involuntary, is a miracle. Each breath you take. Every blink of your eyes. Each beat of your heart. Every time you move your finger or think a thought or hear music or read a book or walk across a room or speak to a neighbor or any one of the millions of actions you take every day of your life involves countless little precision miracles occurring in perfect synchronization within your mind and body.

As mentioned earlier, your body's immune system has been fighting cancer and who-knows-how-many other would-be invaders every minute of your life, and it has done an outstanding job. Another miracle! Abnormal cell division has been triggered time and again throughout your lifetime, but your immune system kicked in and shut it down.

Had you not had a healthy and alert immune system, you might have died from the very first cold or flu virus you encountered as an infant. You might not have recovered from the strep infection you had as a child. That sprained ankle you got playing softball might never have healed. It is quite possible you would not have survived infancy, much less your early childhood.

So your immune system has served you well all of your life until, for one reason or another, it developed a chink in its armor. Maybe it had been weakened over time by a genetic predisposition or environmental factors or lifestyle habits. It doesn't matter now. Whatever the reason, abnormal cell division began, your immune system didn't have the proper defense, and cancer began to grow. That *doesn't* mean your immune system is no longer working, and it certainly doesn't mean that it won't rev up to full speed again. It only means that your body and its immune system need some additional supports *right now*. You and your amazing body are still miracles, and they are going to do many more miraculous things! Just wait and see. You are going to be astounded and amazed at the miracles you are going to be a part of and witness to. You can't and won't do them alone, of course, but you will be an instrumental and absolutely essential participant in the miraculous final result.

Because you are a miracle, you are going to be able to take many, many steps on your own to increase substantially your chances of overcoming cancer. The complicated details will be left to your medical team, but never doubt for a minute that there are lots of very simple actions you can and must take that will greatly improve your odds of a full recovery.

Once we move past the shock of diagnosis (and if you're still in that place, I assure you that, yes, you will move past it), we can then use the time we must spend in treatment to examine what all of this means in our lives. Many cancer survivors have called it "getting your priorities straight" or "gaining new perspective." Roger and I just say we finally "got it."

Cancer does have meaning just as everything in our lives has meaning. We don't grow and learn during the good times. Our characters don't develop and we don't become better, stronger people when times are easy and sweet. It's just the opposite!

We grow bigger and better and stronger when we encounter the worst of times. We become stronger in the places where we have been broken if we allow those places to heal.

Most important, we learn that difficult days and horrible circumstances and painful tragedies and harsh realities are only seasons of our lives, the chilling falls and bitter winters. The happy times – the joyful weddings and births and promotions and holidays and family and friends – are the glorious springs and lush summers.

Kahlil Gibran put this idea into simple, yet eloquent words: "Your pain is the breaking of the shell that encloses your understanding. Even as the stone of the fruit must break that its heart may stand in the sun, so must you know pain. And could you keep your heart in wonder at the daily miracles of your life, your pain would not seem less wondrous than your joy. And you would accept the seasons of your heart, even as you have always accepted the seasons that pass over your fields. And you would watch with serenity through the winters of your grief."

So accept that your life is a miracle and that it moves in a cycle of seasons just as the earth and all living things do. Cancer is one of the dark seasons, but try to do as Gibran so wisely advised. Take a step back and look at the whole of your life. If you will do this, you will see that you will move through this time, and the golden seasons will come again. If you can accept this philosophy, you will find the dark seasons much easier to bear.

Cancer is now a part of your life – whether you are recently diagnosed, a long-term survivor or a caregiver – but your life is no less a miracle for its passing under this cloud. In fact, because you are here now, in this minute, reading this and resolving to learn from the cancer experience and allow it to mold you into a deeper, richer, stronger person than you were before – because of these things, you will emerge from this season as a shining example to all those who will follow you. And yet another miracle will have occurred because of you!

We need to explore and accept some other truths before we move on.

Shortly after my cancer diagnosis, I went to a "healing service" at a local church. I was so desperate and in such a state of panic and anxiety that I was reaching out for anything and everything offered by anyone anywhere at any time. I had no one to guide me through the early stages of coming to terms with my diagnosis. I had no book like this one!

So I went to this healing service with an hysterical kind of joy in my heart thinking that I would leave the church cured of my disease.

During the service, the priest laid his hands on the heads of those who came forward for healing, made the sign of the cross on our foreheads, blessed us and prayed for our healing. But he made it very clear in his prayers and in his homily that, even though we were asking for a return to good health, we understood and accepted that that might not be His will for us. That understood and accepted, then, we were praying for wisdom and understanding of our conditions, strength and courage to face whatever lay ahead, and to be brought into His presence should we not physically survive our diseases.

The priest finished the service with these words: "Sometimes God makes us well. And sometimes He makes us perfect."

"What?" I wondered angrily as I left the church. "What kind of healing service was that? I came here to be healed of my cancer, and all he said was that I might get well and I might not!"

I felt cheated. I wanted so badly for someone – anyone! – to take me by the hand, look me in the eye, and say, "Don't worry. You and Roger will be cured of your cancers and you will live to be 92, give or take a few."

Many of you who are reading this are much wiser and further along your spiritual paths than we were at that time, but I'm including this for those of you who find yourself in that same dark place we were in ten years ago.

There is one overriding truth that we must all accept sooner or later. For us it was later, and it took our simultaneous battles with the beast called cancer to get this truth through our hard heads.

That truth is that there are no guarantees. No one can tell you with 100% certainty that you will survive your disease. And you will be doing yourself a huge favor if you can stop asking them to.

You can slam the book shut now if you feel cheated like I did after the Sunday healing service, but you will come back to this place eventually. Of that I'm sure, and if you need to take some time between now and then, that's okay.

When you're ready, we can move a little further down this road.

The whole truth is that there have been no guarantees from the moment of your conception. There was no guarantee your mother would carry you to full term or that you would be born alive. And from that moment to this, there has never been a single day of your life that anyone could have given you a guarantee in the morning that you would still be there that night.

When Roger was given 50/50 odds of surviving the first year after his diagnosis, he actually said, "I don't think my chances are that good if I get on the interstate to drive home or if we go to the mall on Saturday night." Perhaps a slight exaggeration, but he made a good point!

Once you are able to accept this admittedly unhappy truth ("unhappy" because – let's be honest here – we'd all love to have guarantees of long and healthy lives, and our doctors would love to be able to give them to us), you can move on to the much happier truth.

No one can tell you with 100% certainty that you will not survive your disease either!

Statistics are only indicators of probabilities. They prove *nothing* when we are talking about an individual's odds of surviving a specific illness. Stop asking your doctor and your friend who's a nurse and your nephew who's in medical school and everyone else you think has the inside scoop what they think your chances of surviving your disease are. Don't go online and research graphs and charts, don't read medical textbooks, don't, don't, don't!

Because here's what will happen if you do. If the numbers are bad, your hopefulness will take a little backslide at best; at worst, you'll throw in the towel. If the numbers are good (say, 85% of those diagnosed with your cancer's type and stage survive 5 years), you will at first be elated, but inevitably your mind will find its way back to that 15%, and you will begin wondering who those 15% are and what you might have in common with them that will cause you to join their ranks.

See? Leave the statistics alone. Let the researchers and the doctors and the scientists use them for whatever it is they do with them. You don't need them for anything. They serve no purpose for you whatsoever.

That said, here is the best truth of all, and we've come full circle. Your life is still a miracle! And every single day from now on is going to be a miracle, too.

Accepting that there are no guarantees is life is very freeing. It means that you have confronted the barrier of your mortality, and you have *climbed over it*. Now you are ready to move on to your life beyond your cancer diagnosis – disregarding whether that might mean 2 months or 2 years or 20 years – and allow the Great Physician to complete the miracle He started when He created you.

But you have a huge role to play and lots of work to do. He needs your willingness and cooperation and dedication to the task at hand.

CHAPTER 12

The First 9 of the 10 Things You Absolutely Must Do When the Doctor Says It's Cancer

What follows is a brief and very simple guide to some actions you must take when the doctor says it's cancer. Know that there are countless books and informative websites on each and every one of these important healing steps. All it will take to find books on each topic is a visit to your library or bookstore. Type the subject into the search box of your web browser, and you will find an overwhelming number of websites. Be careful when you are searching the internet, however. As you may already know, anyone can post "information" on the web, and much of it is misleading or just plain wrong. Conduct your research carefully by typing into the search box of your web browser the names of experts and organizations you know you can trust such as the American Cancer Society (www.cancer.org), Dr. Bernie Siegel (www.ecap-online.org) and the American Lung Association (www.lungusa.org).

Grieve

If you have recently been diagnosed with cancer, it's likely you are already grieving. To say that this is a dark and painful place to be would be the greatest understatement we could make. But the only way through this step is a step at a time, one day after another, sometimes taking it minute by minute. We hope that reading this section will help you understand that you are not alone – there are millions of us grieving with you as we grieve our own diagnoses – and also that this is something you just have to move through to get to the other side. There is no way over, under or around it – the only way to the other side is *through*. Just keep telling yourself that you *will* get through this step, and you will move on to the next one and the next one until you come out in a brighter, easier place where you will be much better able to cope, hope and even smile and laugh again.

Okay. Here we go.

Suffering and disease are universal. They affect everyone at some time or another. No one is immune to pain and tragedy and heartache, and no one gets off this planet alive.

Isn't it odd that so many of us spend most of our lives knowing in some far, dark corner of our minds that we are going to die one day, but we keep the door to that place firmly shut so we don't have to look at the reality behind it? Then one day, with little or no warning, the door is thrown open and we are shocked and horrified by the thing we knew all along was there – the simple fact that we are but mere mortals who will one day die.

We're not suggesting for one minute that a diagnosis of cancer means that you are going to die anytime soon! All we are saying is that cancer brings us right up to the brick wall of our mortality. Confronting this wall for the first time is huge, the ultimate reality check, and we have to find a way to get beyond it so that it doesn't become a permanent barrier to our healing.

That is why we must take time to grieve. Bear in mind that what we are grieving is the *loss of our ability to deny our mortality* any longer, "our innocence" if you will. We can't shut the door again. It has been thrown open and we have been forced to look the beast in the eye.

I was 45 years old when I was diagnosed, but I dug out the teddy bear I'd had since childhood and curled up in the fetal position in the middle of my bed and cried for three days. A few people tried to make me "snap out of it" (I think the truth is the intensity of my grieving frightened them), and several admonished me to "get a positive attitude" if I was going to "beat this thing," but I know now that they were wrong and I was right because *I was doing what felt right to me at that time.* My instinct was correct: I needed time to grieve. And I needed to do it my way.

Everyone grieves the loss of their health, but not everyone grieves the same way. Give yourself time to grieve in whatever way feels right to you. If others want to interfere and try to redirect your grieving, find a way to remove yourself from them while you do your work (grieving is soul work). Don't allow anyone to tell you not to cry or to "pull yourself together" or "get a grip" or "put on a smile" or any of the other empty bits of so-called advice people who haven't been where you are will offer. The fact of the matter is that they want you to do these things so that you will stop upsetting and frightening them. And this isn't about them, so remove yourself from these people and do what you need to do.

The only exception we would make here would be if you are the parent of young children. If the intensity of your grieving is such that it could be frightening or upsetting to them, find a safe place for you to go where you can do your grieving without their having to watch, or allow them to go off on a cheerful weekend visit with relatives or friends. We did the latter and, while it was not a perfect solution, it was far better than allowing them to see us in the state we were in. They would eventually have to know that both of their parents had cancer, but that bombshell had to wait until Roger and I composed ourselves enough to explain it to them in terms they could understand and without unduly frightening them.

One newly diagnosed friend of mine was so bombarded by people trying to cheer her up and keep her from crying and so worried about her young daughter witnessing the intensity of her grief that she packed a bag and went to a rented cottage at the beach. Her daughter went to visit her grandmother for the week. It was the off season, and the beach community was practically deserted. My friend was able to spend several days walking by the ocean, pitching pebbles and shells into the water, alternately shaking her fists and screaming her anger at God (don't worry if you want to do this, too; He can handle it), then falling to her knees in the sand, praying and asking Him to embrace and heal her, crying until her tears were all cried out, and finally sleeping around the clock for two days. She returned home, exhausted yet relieved, her grief work done. She was ready to face the surgeries and treatments that lay ahead, and she was ready to help her daughter through the difficult days to come.

You may find it helpful to track your grieving through the seven stages of grief as defined by Elisabeth Kubler-Ross. She noted these stages are shock, denial, bargaining, guilt, anger, depression and acceptance.

You probably don't need any explanation of the shock part of this picture – by the time you're reading this book, you've most likely been there and done that.

You may already have experienced some denial. You may have told yourself that your test results must have been mixed up with someone else's. The pathologist made a mistake. The radiologist saw some scar tissue from the appendectomy you had when you were twelve and thought he was looking at a tumor.

We all play these games to some extent, and as we've already said, it's a natural stage of grieving. Denial is the mind's way of cushioning the blow as it comes out of the shock stage, and it is the mind's way of very gradually beginning to consider the information it has to absorb.

You finally realize that the diagnosis is real and it is yours. You may enter into a period of bargaining with God. "If You will just take this cancer away, I promise I will be a better person. I'll do volunteer work. I'll sell everything I own and give all the money to charity. I'll do *anything*, just please, please take this cancer away."

It doesn't take us long to realize that bargaining isn't going to accomplish a cure. So we move on to guilt.

This is a stage where you can really and needlessly torture yourself if you're not careful, so we want to encourage you to try hard to get past it as quickly as possible. The fact of the matter is that guilt serves no purpose whatsoever when we're talking about a diagnosis of cancer. Nobody knows why you got cancer, and more importantly, it doesn't matter now.

Later we'll talk about some of the things you will want to start doing and some other things you will want to stop doing in order to maximize the success potential of your treatment and minimize the risk of disease recurrence, but that doesn't mean you should feel guilty about having done or not done those same things in the past. Remember, we're only looking to the future now. We can learn from the past and use what we learn to create a better future, but we can't change the past. Let it go.

Now we get to the two that are, in my opinion, the toughest. Not necessarily the toughest to get through (for me, that was the shock phase), but the hardest to let go of.

Nothing could be more natural in the face of a diagnosis of cancer than anger. You have a right to be mad. Furious, in fact. There is nothing fair about this disease. It is completely indiscriminate, attacking the innocent and the evil alike, although sometimes it seems it mostly attacks the best and the brightest, the tiniest and most innocent, the sweetest and most vulnerable.

Go ahead and get mad, but *let the anger out.* Don't sit around and seethe. Letting it build up inside you and holding it in is unhealthy. Do something physically active to release the anger. Pound your fists into a pillow. Beat your mattress with a tennis racket. Throw rocks in a lake or ocean. Break some eggs in the sink or bathtub. If, like many newly diagnosed cancer patients, you're otherwise strong and healthy, take a brisk walk or a bike ride.

These are just suggestions. You'll think of the right thing for you. Take any kind of physical action you are capable of taking to rid your body of the angry feelings. Whatever you choose to do, do it until you've exhausted the anger.

When you have exhausted the anger, chances are you will enter a stage of mild-to-moderate depression from which you will emerge fairly quickly (several weeks to a few months for most people), moving on to the stage of acceptance (the real beginning of the healing process!).

For a few, however, and as it was for me, this was the hardest and longest lasting stage. Today I know it didn't have to be that way, and I don't want it to be that way for you.

As you move through each of the stages of grief, it's important to communicate with your doctor and let him know where you are. He will want to know that you are moving through the process and not getting "stuck" at any one stage. If you do get stuck, he will know what to do to help you get "unstuck."

But at no time is this careful self-observation and open communication more important than when you are in a state of depression. Many newly diagnosed cancer patients need additional support during this time. I did, but I wasn't self-aware enough to realize it.

Some people are able to step outside themselves, so to speak, and observe themselves as others are seeing them. A deeply depressed person will not be able to do this, however, and it will be up to family members and friends to ask the following questions: Is the patient sleeping much more or much less than normal? Is he refusing to get out of bed even though he is physically able? Has she stopped eating, or is she eating constantly? Is he unable to stop crying? Has she stopped bathing, brushing her teeth, getting dressed, combing her hair? Is he self-medicating with alcohol and/or illegal drugs? Has she talked about deliberately ending her life?

These are signs of serious depression that require immediate medical intervention. If you recognize these symptoms in yourself, or if you are a family member of friend of a newly diagnosed cancer patient and you observe these behaviors in the patient, please contact the patient's physician right away. It may be that medication is needed or "talk therapy" or a combination of the two, but whatever is required, the patient's doctor is the one who needs to make those decisions, and he can't help the patient if he isn't aware of the problem. Please make him aware of the problem so that the patient can move on to the stage of acceptance and begin the work of healing.

And finally we arrive at the stage of acceptance. *Acceptance does not mean surrender. Repeat: Acceptance does not mean surrender!*

Acceptance simply means that we have gotten past the negativity, rid ourselves of feelings of anger and defeat, stopped feeling guilty, quit trying to deny or bargain, moved through the depression and arrived at a place where we can begin to heal.

Believe it or not, we have known cancer patients who have moved through all seven of these stages in a day or two! Some have only needed a week or two! I am amazed and inspired by these people and wish like heck I could be like them, but that's just not my emotional make-up. *You* just might turn out to be one of these people, though, and if you are, Roger and I are really happy for you! If you're like us, though, and find yourself moving slowly through the stages, be very sure to surround yourself with supportive family members and friends. Ask them to help you move through the stages and to observe you and to let you and your doctor know if they think you're becoming "stuck."

Breathe!

When we panic or remain in a heightened state of anxiety for a period of time, we tend to take rapid, shallow breaths. The longer we breathe this way, the more our panic and anxiety can increase, and we can even experience dizziness and fainting due to hyperventilation.

Become aware of your breathing. Slow it down.

Practice the following deep breathing exercise: Sit in a comfortable chair and focus on relaxing every muscle in your body, beginning with your facial muscles and working your way slowly down to your toes. When your entire body is relaxed and comfortable, place one hand lightly on your midsection with the tip of your little finger on your navel. This puts your hand directly over your diaphragm. Begin to inhale deeply through your nose, concentrating on making your hand rise, filling your diaphragm first, then continuing to inhale and filling your lungs and chest last. Count slowly to four as you breathe in. Then hold the breath and count slowly to four again. Begin to exhale slowly through your mouth, emptying your chest and lungs first, working your way back down to your diaphragm. If you find that a count of 5 or 6 or 8 works better for you, that's fine. Just be sure that the count is the same for the inhale, hold and exhale. Repeat 5 times.

Practice this exercise throughout the day, as often as you think about it. If you have trouble remembering to do it, write yourself a note or set an alarm on your watch or cell phone or oven timer. Find a way to remind yourself to do this exercise. After a while, slow, deep breathing will become second nature to you, enhancing your mental clarity, helping you conserve your strength, increasing your energy level and helping you sleep better. You will feel calmer and better able to cope with the challenges of your diagnosis and treatment.

There is something else we are talking about, however, when we remind newly diagnosed cancer survivors to breathe. We are talking about "taking a breather."

In other words, call a temporary halt to everything if it seems like it's all just spinning out of control. Just stop.

The first hours, days and weeks after a cancer diagnosis are frantic for most. You have a million questions. You're frightened. There are so many decisions to make about your family and your work. There's so much to learn. You may have more medical appointments in the next few months than you've had in your entire life. There are treatment decisions that you have to make, decisions that can affect the rest of your life, and you don't even know enough about any of it to make any decisions!

This is when you need to stop and take a deep breath, literally and figuratively. *You have time* to learn about your disease, request a second and third opinion, explore treatment options and make decisions. When you feel yourself becoming panicky and your anxiety level shooting through the roof, take a time out. Chances are, nothing has to be decided today.

Talk it over with your doctor. He may tell you that your surgery decision can wait another few days. He may tell you that your chemotherapy treatments can begin after your vacation or after the holidays. He may tell you a particular medication regimen can wait until after your big birthday celebration. The important thing is to discuss it with your doctor and open up to him about your concerns and fears. He will almost certainly have some solutions and options for you to consider that will have you feeling calmer and more in control right away.

Insist on an immediate referral to a medical oncologist.

One of the biggest mistakes we made when Roger was diagnosed with cancer was that we did not ask for a referral to a medical oncologist (a medical doctor who specializes in cancer diagnosis and treatment). At that point, we simply didn't know to ask.

It wasn't until several months later when I sat down for the first time with the medical oncologist to whom I had been referred as a result of *my* cancer diagnosis that Roger had an opportunity to ask questions about *his* diagnosis. The medical oncologist thoroughly and compassionately answered both of our questions about both of our cases over the course of two hours. He was able to relieve worries that had troubled us about Roger's diagnosis for nearly three months, worries that could have been eased considerably when he was first diagnosed had we known to ask for a referral to a medical oncologist.

Don't accept an answer of "It's too soon" or "It isn't necessary." We know of cases where compassionate family doctors have made a referral to a medical oncologist even before a biopsy has been performed or any definitive diagnosis made.

You have a right to talk to the person who is most knowledgeable about your disease. In the case of most cancer diagnoses, that person is a medical oncologist.

Insist.

And while we're on the subject of doctors, there is a good chance that you will have a medical team made up of at least several doctors. My team was made up of a surgeon, a medical oncologist, a radiation oncologist (all doctors, of course) and five or six nurses and technicians. No matter how many medical professionals you may end up working with, do not allow yourself to become a name on a chart to any of them. Don't be passive, submissive, quiet and shy, thinking you will fare better if you don't make waves. Be the patient who asks questions and takes notes. Be the patient who shows pictures of his wife and kids. Be the patient who insists her doctors meet her family and see her new grandchild. Invite the doctor out to the parking lot to see your new car. Send your treatment nurses a fruit basket. If you're the creative type, create something for the doctor's office. Send holiday cards to your medical team. Share jokes with them.

Above all, insist that they talk to you and treat you like the most important patient they have ever had because, you know what? You *are* the most important patient they have ever had, and so is every patient they treat. Sometimes they are overworked and they get tired, and they forget this. Don't let them forget it on your time.

A friend of mine was being prepped for her first chemotherapy treatment, and she asked the treatment nurse why a certain procedure was being done. The nurse responded that it made it easier for her (the nurse) to administer my friend's treatment. My friend politely but firmly explained to the nurse that, while what she said may have been true, it hadn't been necessary to explain it quite that way to a patient. Cancer treatment should never be about what is "easiest" for the treatment team. It should always be about what is best for the patient's physical, emotional, mental and spiritual well-being. Sometimes the professionals need to be reminded of that.

Stop doing the things you know you are not supposed to be doing.

You might be amazed at the number of times we have seen cancer survivors step outside of treatment centers and light up cigarettes. Then again, this might be you!

You might be surprised to learn that many newly diagnosed cancer patients eat nothing but high-fat fast foods and junk foods. Sound familiar?

You might be dumbfounded to know that some patients show up for surgeries or other treatments under the influence of alcohol and/or illegal drugs. And some patients don't show up for their surgeries or treatments at all.

The world renowned author and motivational speaker Zig Ziglar uses the following hypothetical situation to make this point: If you owned a million-dollar thoroughbred racehorse, would you allow it to be exposed to toxic substances like cigarette smoke? Would you feed it cookies and chips and soda? Would you let it stay out all night in the pasture, carousing with its horsey friends? Would you give it alcohol or illegal substances?

Of course not! You'd make sure it breathed clean air, ate only the finest, most nutritious feed, exercised and grazed by day and rested snug in its stall at night, and never ever ate or drank anything that wasn't beneficial to its overall health and well-being.

You are not a million-dollar thoroughbred racehorse. You are a billion-dollar-plus human being with unlimited potential. Why, oh, why would you do any less for yourself?

If you are doing anything to your body that is negative in any way, that is in any way not healthful and helpful, now is the time to stop.

Start doing the things you know you are supposed to be doing.

Resolve right now – this minute – to make the positive lifestyle changes you know will improve your chances of a longer, healthier life. Whatever the current status of your health – whether you are a cancer patient or healthy caregiver – you can absolutely improve the quality of your life and probably extend its length by making some lifestyle changes right now.

1. Drink water. Everyone needs to drink six to eight 8-ounce glasses of water a day. Cancer patients especially need to stay well hydrated. Drinking plenty of water reduces the severity of some side effects and can prevent others. Staying well hydrated plumps up veins and makes infusions and blood draws easier. Drinking plenty of water flushes toxins from your body. And drink *clean* water. When a plumbing problem in our neighborhood prompted the city to replace some pipes that went from the street into the homes, we were appalled at the corrosion and build-up of God-only-knows-

what in those fifty-year old pipes. We had been drinking water that came through those nasty pipes for years. We quickly contracted with a local company (as did all of our neighbors) to have bottled distilled water delivered to our house every week. You might want to consider this option.

2. Drink tea. And don't let anyone tell you it has to be green tea. Green tea and black tea (the standard varieties and brands of grocery store tea you've always used for hot and iced tea) are very high in antioxidants (remember, they're the "good guys" that scavenge free radicals which are the "bad buys" that can cause cancer) and they're about equal. In addition to being a powerful cancer fighter, tea has also been proven to lower bad cholesterol and protect bones and teeth. Make your own rather than buying bottled tea as some antioxidants found in tea tend to break down over time. Herbal teas may be good for some other conditions and symptoms, but when we're talking about powerful cancer fighting agents, we're talking about black and green teas.

3. "Eat the rainbow." Choose most of the foods you eat from plant sources, and eat nine servings of fruits and vegetables a day. That's right, *nine* – not five. The standard recommendation has been five, but there are some studies that indicate that anyone who has had a diagnosis of cancer needs to up that number to nine. Go heavy on the vegetables, too, meaning five vegetables and four fruits, not the other way around. Fruits and vegetables contain essential vitamins, minerals, fiber and antioxidants, all of which have been proven to significantly reduce cancer risk and strengthen your immune system so that you are better able to withstand and battle illness. The more colorful the fruit or vegetable, the more nutrition it packs, so eat a wide variety of colors and textures – keep the rainbow in mind when shopping the produce aisles. And don't think you have to eat huge portions to reap the benefits. Healthy portions are relatively small: ½ cup of fruit or 1 medium piece of fruit, ¼ cup of dried fruit, ¾ cup of 100% fruit or vegetable

juice, 1 cup of leafy vegetables, ½ cup of cooked or raw vegetables. Frozen vegetables are every bit as nutritious as fresh, so don't let the seasons control your menu choices. Buy organic fruits and vegetables whenever possible, and thoroughly wash all produce with the produce washes now available in most supermarkets. Eat only whole grain cereals, breads, pastas and other grain products. Avoid white flour and sugar.

4. Cut way back on red meat. Avoid it altogether if you can. Choose turkey and chicken from farmers who don't inject their animals with growth hormones and antibiotics. I cornered my doctor on this one. I asked him about red meat after reading several reports about increased cancer risks caused by growth hormones and antibiotics administered to most beef cattle and some chickens and turkeys in this country. The doctor made vague, mostly unresponsive comments to the effect that "nothing has really been proven." Then I asked him, "Do you eat red meat?" His answer? An unqualified "No!" Eat fish. If you don't care for fish, take a daily fish oil supplement. Eat beans.

5. Get busy. We've all heard that walking is the safest, easiest and most effective of all physical activities, and it certainly carries the least risk of injury. This popular form of exercise has even been shown to reduce anxiety and mild-to-moderate depression. We vote for walking as the ideal exercise for most people. Thirty minutes of walking every day is an exercise program that even the most un-athletic among us can live with, and even most cancer patients currently undergoing treatment can enjoy a walk. When you have finished your treatments and had time to recover your strength, and with your doctor's blessing, consider adding other activities to your exercise program. The possibilities are endless. Remember how you loved to ride your bike or roller skate as a kid? Enjoy a favorite childhood activity again. Were you a track star or tennis champion in high school? Believe it or not, it's not too late to return to the sports you loved when you were younger and stronger.

It's not even too late to win medals and trophies again. Two words: Lance Armstrong. We don't even pretend to think that we're in the same league with Lance, but we did complete an amazing athletic feat four years after being diagnosed with cancer, enduring lengthy and aggressive treatments, and receiving "iffy" prognoses. If two extremely ill, middle-aged, overweight and out-of-shape former smokers like us can do what we did, then there's hope for everyone. Never, never, never give up. No matter how bad you feel today, you have to believe that tomorrow will be better. And the next day will be even better than the one before. Join the YMCA or a fitness center and take a class in anything from spinning to yoga. Too self-conscious to work out in public? Work out in the privacy of your own home with a treadmill and/or exercise videos.

6. Maintain a healthy weight. Roger and I struggle with this one daily, but it's always foremost in our minds and we are always working on it. Excess weight has been linked to numerous medical conditions and diseases including cancers of the breast, uterus and colon. If you're overweight, make losing the extra pounds a priority. Following the nutrition and exercise guidelines above will help bring your weight into the healthy range and keep it there. If you are already at a healthy weight, strive to maintain it. Weight gain and loss are difficult issues for cancer patients. Chemotherapy treatments can cause loss of appetite resulting in weight loss. On the other hand, some treatments can actually make you gain unwanted weight! If you're experiencing cancer-related weight concerns, be sure to consult with your physician. She knows how important it is to maintain a healthy weight and can provide nutrition counseling and other support.

7. You booze, you lose. While it is true that some studies have shown a glass of red wine or beer to have certain health benefits, the potential risks of overindulging in "adult beverages" far outweigh any possible good they may do. Recent studies point to an increased cancer risk for women who average one drink a day or more and

in men who average two drinks a day or more. Alcohol increases the risk of cancers of the colon, esophagus, breast, mouth and throat. If you do drink, drink in moderation. Consider not drinking at all.

8. Wear sunscreen and, as much as possible, avoid outdoor activities when the sun is at its highest. Children six months of age and older should be protected by sunscreen any time they are outdoors. Babies under six months of age should not wear sunscreen, but should be shielded from the sun by their clothing and by hoods or visors over their strollers. Wear hats and sunglasses.

9. Avoid vehicle exhaust fumes and the fumes from gasoline when fueling your car or lawn equipment. Choose pest control companies that use organic materials, or purchase electronic devices from a home improvement store. Avoid exposure to known carcinogens used in many industries such as asbestos, vinyl chloride, chromate and nickel, to name just a few. Keep a watchful eye on the industries in your community. Find out what's in the black smoke being belched from that smokestack across town. Find out what that smell is that's in the air every Tuesday and Thursday morning. Have your water analyzed. Advocate for legislation to ensure clean air and water where you live.

10. Get plenty of rest and restful sleep. It is very common for cancer patients to have trouble sleeping, but getting enough restful sleep is one of the most essential steps toward healing. Please don't hesitate to ask your doctor for a prescription sleep aid during this difficult time. If you follow his instructions carefully and responsibly, you will *not* become an "addict" as so many patients worry about. You *will* be less depressed and better able to tolerate your treatments and cope with all of the circumstances of your diagnosis if you are well rested. Believe me, your doctor wants and needs you to be well rested. So tell him if you need some help in this (or any other, such as loss of appetite) area.

Avoid self-medicating.

Many cancer patients are tempted to rush to the health food store and start taking every nutritional "supplement" and vitamin on the shelves. *Don't do it.* Talk to your doctor and ask what vitamins and/or supplements, if any, he recommends.

Here's why. Certain supplements, herbal "remedies" and "natural cures" can actually interfere with your medical treatments. For example, St. John's Wort's has been proven in several studies to help some patients with mild-to-moderate depression, *but it has also been proven to interfere with the efficacy of a widely prescribed anti-cancer drug!* And some medical professionals question the safety of the use of soy products by women with some breast cancers, even though soy products have been shown to be beneficial for the general population.

The bottom line is that only your medical team knows the details of your treatment plan and the chemistry of the drugs you are taking and all of the myriad bits of information about you and your body that need to be taken into consideration before adding anything else to the mix. You may be the captain of the team, but your doctor is the head coach with all the knowledge, skills and experience needed to make important decisions about what goes into your body during your treatment for cancer. This includes over-the-counter medications, too, such as pain relievers and cold and flu medications.

If there is a certain supplement you want to try, ask the doctor first. Chances are he will say, "Can't hurt. Go ahead." But far better to be safe than sorry.

About that positive attitude thing...

Don't groan! And don't be alarmed if it takes you quite a while to "arrive" at a positive attitude. A cancer diagnosis can knock the most optimistic Pollyanna among us to her knees. It's okay. Once you've had time to work through those stages of grieving we talked about before, you'll be ready to start working on a brighter outlook, and that's soon enough. Above all, be gentle with yourself and give yourself time.

Now, once you're ready, how do you go about it? Well, there are actually quite a few very specific things you can do to improve your outlook and develop an I-can-do-this attitude.

As mentioned earlier, don't look for or listen to statistics and "time limits." The fact is that somebody has beaten every kind of cancer there is! There are survivors of every type and stage of this disease. No one – not even your doctor – has all the answers or can tell you with certainty what the outcome of your diagnosis and treatment will be. The best they can do is venture an educated guess, and whether it's positive or negative, a guess isn't going to do you any good at all, so best to just leave it alone. You have far more important things to do. So go forth and do these things.

Stay connected to friends and family. They're struggling with your diagnosis, too. Allow them to care for you. Giving and receiving care are healing for the giver and the receiver.

On the other hand, if you find that certain people can only be negative around you and want to tell you cancer horror stories, avoid them for the time being. For some unknown reason, a couple of people insisted on calling me after hearing I'd been diagnosed with breast cancer just to tell me about their Great Aunt Betty or Cousin Flo who "died of the very same thing." What were they thinking? These conversations brought me so low at a time when I didn't think I could feel any lower! I mentioned this to my doctor during an appointment, and he did two very important things. First, he told me that it is quite likely that Great Aunt Betty and Cousin Flo died ten or more years ago (I hadn't thought to ask), before there were so many wonderful treatment options available *and* that nobody has ever had the "very same thing" I had because every case is different in so many ways that lay people like us have no business whatsoever making such comparisons.

He then instructed Roger to "run interference" for me. Roger began answering the door and the telephone and letting everyone who wanted to talk to me know in no uncertain terms that they had better be upbeat and only share stories with happy endings with me or their visits and calls would no longer be welcome! This is an important part of taking care of yourself – don't ignore it. Surround yourself with positive, cheerful people, and ask your caregivers to keep all others away!

This next one may seem a little far out, but stay with me here. *Wear clothes that make you feel braver and stronger or that make you feel good or that make you or those around you laugh.* I learned the power of this one day when I was getting ready to go to the clinic for my chemotherapy treatment. I was scrounging around for something to wear, and threw on my son's "No Fear" brand t-shirt. When I got to the clinic, a couple of other patients commented on my shirt. "That's the attitude!" said one. "You tell 'em!" said another. My mood brightened, and suddenly I felt braver and stronger because of a few words on a t-shirt!

I started wearing shirts and ball caps that had the logos of the Army, the Marine Corps, a local fire department and the regional police academy. When I was wearing these items, I found that I felt like part of a bigger team of strong, powerful people. I adopted a "warrior mentality" and began to carry that image of myself in my head: me as a soldier fighting for my life and winning.

I started looking for shirts that had statements on them about courage and endurance and strength. I also made sure I wore bright colors, and sometimes I wore shirts and hats that were funny so I could make others laugh. I found that my mood mirrored what I wore!

On good days, I put on make-up and either styled my wig or wore a pretty turban, and I put on colorful, pretty clothes.

On bad days, this was a challenge, and on really bad days, I just didn't worry about my appearance at all. There may be times like that for you, when just focusing on getting through the day is all you can handle, and that's fine. Again, be gentle with yourself. If worrying about your appearance only adds to your fatigue and discomfort, let it go. But when you're feeling well enough and energetic enough to put some effort into how you look, know that the clothes you wear, a little make-up (or a shave for you guys) and a flattering head covering can lift your spirits even higher.

Create and practice comforting rituals. At times of crisis and upheaval in our lives, it helps to stick to familiar routines as much as possible. We can find added comfort, however, by including comforting rituals to our daily schedules. Set aside time to brew a pot of tea, soak in a warm bath, rest while listening to a CD of a rain shower or ocean waves, light a candle and meditate or pray. Rituals are calming and restorative. Create your own and make them a part of your daily healing.

Celebrate every milestone. Stitches out today? Celebrate! Last chemotherapy or radiation treatment? Celebrate! First hair coming back in? For gosh sakes, celebrate! Whatever your favorite means of celebrating, do it. Go out to dinner. Buy a new outfit. Go away for the weekend. Have friends over. Do it up big or keep it small, but whatever you do, celebrate!

Remember that humor heals. Go to the website of the American Film Institute (www.afi.com) and follow the links to their listing of the 100 funniest movies ever made. Then start working your way through the list. Watch, read and listen to funny tapes, books and CDs. Watch sit-coms and those "funniest videos" specials on TV. Likewise, avoid scary, sad or violent movies and books. Not only are you what you eat; you are also what you read and observe.

Give a kitten a piece of ribbon or blow bubbles for a puppy. Play peek-a-boo with a toddler. Do whatever makes you laugh. Do it every day.

There is even a school of thought that advocates making yourself laugh even when – no, especially when – you don't feel like it. Don't wait for something funny, these folks say. Pretend you are an actor on stage and the script calls for you to laugh long and hard. Then do it. This is the fake-it-'til-you-can-make-it line of thinking, and it really does work. After a few tries, you will find that your mood responds to your body's laughter.

Utilize positive visualizations. Use the breathing exercise described earlier to bring yourself into a calm, relaxed state. With your eyes closed and your breathing slow and steady, create a mental picture of yourself as a strong, healthy survivor. Take that image through whatever experience represents for you the achievement of your goal. See yourself strong and well, robust and healthy, a long-term cancer survivor enjoying life to the fullest, engaged in activities you enjoy, surrounded by loved ones, laughing and joyful.

Savor pleasurable things. Be fully aware and mindful – *be in the moment* – when you are engaged in an activity that gives you pleasure. Eating the last watermelon in summer or the first apple of fall. Watching a storm or a sunset. Dancing with someone you love. Reading a novel. Building a model ship. Whatever gives you pleasure – as long as it's legal and doesn't interfere with your treatment! – do it and savor every moment.

Keep a joy journal.

We encourage cancer patients to keep a journal for many reasons, not the least of which is the simple fact that this is an incredibly difficult part of your life journey and, whether you realize it right now or not, you are growing and changing into a different person – a better person in many ways – than the person you were before your diagnosis. The day will come when you will want to look back over this experience and consider all that you learned from it and even the many blessings you received as a result. Keeping a journal now will help you recall circumstances, events, people and details that your memory won't hold onto.

Keeping a journal will also help you remember questions you want to ask your doctor, symptoms that were here one day and gone the next that you need to mention to her; too, it will give you a visual readout of your good days and bad days so that you have a better idea when one or the other is coming and can be prepared for it.

But most of all, we encourage patients to keep a journal and to record joy in it every single day. You will have to look harder for joy on some days than on others, but if you look hard enough, you will find it. Write about a person you encountered who smiled or said something kind or supported you in some way and made you feel better. Write about something you did well. Write about something you like about yourself. Remember a joyful time in your past. Write about activities you enjoyed as a child, and think and write about ways you could enjoy them again. Write about your partner and the things you adore about him or her. Write about times when you've felt peaceful and serene. Write about a time when you laughed so hard you cried or milk came out of your nose. Write about someone you want to forgive. Write a thank you note to God. Count your blessings and write them down.

Do your spiritual homework.

We would never dream of telling anyone what their "spiritual homework" is because it's different for every individual. You may have been raised in a family that had strong religious ties to one faith, or you may have grown up in an environment that didn't put a lot of emphasis on religion. Whatever your spiritual or cultural background and beliefs, now is the time to explore and practice them.

If you've never had any at all or if the ones you grew up with don't feel like a good "fit" now, then this can be an exciting time of exploration of many faiths and cultural beliefs.

You may want to meet with a pastor, priest, rabbi, shaman or other leader/counselor from your own faith or one you want to learn more about. You may recall religious rituals that brought you comfort in the past, lighting a candle in a chapel or singing a favorite hymn or chanting a prayer or blessing. Or you may want to try these things for the first time. Whether you choose to worship in a formal setting or connect with your Higher Power at the beach or on a mountaintop, find a way to make that connection and then make it a part of your everyday life.

Cancer patients who have strong ties to religious and cultural traditions move more easily through their diagnoses and treatments and feel more supported and hopeful overall.

There are countless stories of spontaneous remissions and cures believed to be the results of prayer and for which no other explanations can be found or offered. We are convinced of the validity of many of them and would love to re-tell some of those stories here, but they will have to wait for another book and another time as we need to move on now to the last of the ten things you absolutely must do when the doctor says it's cancer…

CHAPTER 13

Do Something Amazing!

Whether you have realized it yet or not, you have been given a tremendous gift and blessing through your cancer experience. You are more alive in this moment than you ever were before cancer became a part of your life. Everything seems different somehow. Most things seem better. You've gained perspective and you don't sweat the small stuff anymore.

You may even find that you feel sorry for those who just seem to be "going through the motions" of daily life. They don't appear to appreciate the simple things you've come to embrace and treasure, things as majestic as a sunset or rainbow, as achingly beautiful as a baby's laugh or a church choir, as uplifting as a hug from a friend or the gift of a tiny, perfect shell from the ocean. You'd like to think they will someday learn to see things through new eyes like you've been given, but you'd also like to think they can do that without going through what you've endured or something else equally seismic and life-altering.

Chances are they can't. Unfortunately, it usually takes something like a diagnosis of cancer to bring us to this level of awareness and gratitude, but now that you have achieved it, *you must do something with it.*

You have been given the opportunity to get past that wall we spoke of earlier, the wall of your mortality. Once you are beyond that wall, you have not only accepted your mortality, you have come to the understanding that *our mortality is what makes life worth living.* You understand that even the youngest, healthiest and strongest person among us is not guaranteed tomorrow. You embrace that understanding and commit to using it to live each and every day of your life like it's your very last because now you understand that it just could be. And while you may not be exactly okay with that, you know that you've learned and grown enough through this experience that when that day comes, you can and will accept it with grace and dignity because you've had the opportunity to go forward after your diagnosis and treatment and live the life you were meant to live.

That's what we mean when we say, "Do something amazing!"

Do what you know you were born to do.

You might already be doing what you think you were born to do, but chances are you're not, or that, at the very least, your life could be far more fulfilling than it is now.

Every human being was put on this earth for a reason, and each and every one of us was given certain talents and gifts with which to become who and what we are supposed to be. Now is the time to make absolutely certain that you are squeezing every ounce of talent and ability and skill and knowledge out of yourself and using it to saturate every area of your life

You may have enjoyed doing with your life whatever you've been doing up to this point. Doesn't matter what that is. What matters is whether you have ever fantasized about doing something else. Have you wished you had become an actor or a musician or an artist? Have you wanted to study pharmacy or criminal justice or the culture of a primitive population? Ever thought of taking a photographic safari? Climbing a mountain? White water rafting? Learning shorthand? Building a birdhouse, a garage, a web site? Do you love to experiment in the kitchen? In the lab? In the garden? Want to write a book? Produce a play? Compose a musical score? Have you always wished you'd learned to play tennis? Swim? Ice skate?

We could ask hundreds of these questions, but you get the picture.

In his book *Cancer as a Turning Point*, Dr. Lawrence LeShan says, "Our actions are usually based on … 'shoulds' rather than on the question of 'what would fulfill me – what *style* of being, relating, creating would bring me to a life of zest?' This is the life, this life and the search for it, that mobilizes the immune system against cancer more than anything else we know today."

Dr. LeShan cites case after case of cancer patients (many of whom had been led to believe they only had a few months or perhaps years to live) who made complete lifestyle changes so that they began truly living the lives they had always dreamed of living and whose "incurable" cancers went into long, unanticipated and sometimes apparently permanent remissions (many of his patients were still alive and well when Dr. LeShan's book was published, many years out from their original diagnoses and treatments).

That's what Roger and I did. We changed our *style* of being, relating and creating. We changed everything about the way we lived our lives. We believe this is probably the single most powerful survival tool that you can use yourself, and the one that we believe sealed our survival once we had completed our medical treatments.

We changed everything about the way we lived our lives even to the point of redecorating our home, simplifying and de-cluttering, and creating an atmosphere of peace and solitude. We almost always have candles burning, and we listen to soft music or nature sounds or guided imagery tapes and CDs. All of our rooms have diffused lighting and lots of natural light. We have several small table-top fountains and one free-standing floor fountain because we find the sound of rippling water soothing. We have carved out small spaces in our home that are retreats for each of us for prayer and meditation. We bought a new mattress so that our sleep would be more restful. Everywhere in our home are books of inspirational essays, poetry, positive visualizations, meditations and prayers.

We seldom watch television unless there is something of real informational value or artistic merit. Sadly, the nightly news has become little more than a police report; we seldom read our local newspaper for the same reason.

No one is allowed to raise his or her voice in our home. Instead of arguing until somebody "wins," we prefer to agree to disagree. Nothing is important enough to fight over or for except life itself.

We've learned not to jump every time the phone rings. We've learned it's okay to use Caller ID. We've learned that some people are "psychic vampires" who seem to suck all the air out of the room when they enter and who will try to suck all of your hope and joy out of you, and we simply don't invite them into our home; if we encounter them elsewhere, we make a hasty exit.

Are there some changes you can make in your home to make it a more peaceful, healing environment? Now is the time to make those changes.

Earlier in this book, I mentioned that before our cancer diagnoses, I had dreamed of living at the beach and writing romance novels, and Roger longed to become a professional speaker and conduct business seminars. The cancer experience helped us refine those dreams. Today we are *both* professional speakers and we are *both* writers. In addition to helping us gain perspective on what is important in life and what is not, the cancer experience has also given us a mission, and that is to bring a healing message of hope and humor to cancer survivors and caregivers. We are accomplishing that through our speaking and our writing. We are living our dreams, just not in quite the way we had envisioned them before cancer.

We are living more and more of our dreams every day. We haven't moved to the beach yet, but we go there as often as we can, sometimes for a week, sometimes just for a weekend, but we *go*.

I'm working on a novel, but it's not a romance. Remember I said that the cancer experience helped us refine our dreams? Writing a romance, it turned out, was not what I really wanted to do, at least not right now. I really want to write a mainstream novel, and that's what I'm doing.

Roger is creating a series of business seminars and workshops, but that goal has been refined, too. He realized that his favorite aspect of business and the one in which he has the greatest expertise is customer service, and that's what he's focusing on.

The cancer experience will – if you allow it to – bring everything in your life into the sharpest possible focus.

What are your dreams? Are they in sharp focus? Now is the time to refine your dreams. Get very specific with them. *Begin to live them now.*

We've heard so many stories of people who have drastically changed every single aspect of their lives after cancer, and the end result is that they are living the rest of their lives doing what they always knew they wanted to do. A single teacher resigned from her position after being diagnosed with and treated for breast cancer, sold all of her belongings, and joined the Peace Corps. She's still teaching, but she's teaching women and children in a remote African village to raise crops and livestock so they can be self-sufficient. A newspaper editor who was told she would probably die within two years of her cancer diagnosis quit her job, sold everything and moved to a small village in Italy where she studied oil painting with a local artist. This was a fantasy she had held since childhood. She is now a selling artist, living and loving life in the Italian countryside, whose work is in much demand – ten years after she was expected to die.

If these kinds of lifestyle changes seem unrealistic or even impossible to you due to your own life circumstances, I encourage you to write down your wildest dream and the lifestyle changes that would have to occur in order for you to achieve it. Then break it all down into small steps and explore on paper ways in which each step could be taken. It's easy to say, "Oh, I can't follow my dream of _____ because of _____," but if you break it down into "baby steps" and figure out realistic ways in which those steps can be taken, you will be surprised to discover that your fantasy isn't unrealistic at all. Your fantasies and your dreams are your mind's way of telling you what you really want and what you really should be doing. Bear in mind we're talking about career and lifestyle fantasies and dreams here, not bizarre illegal, immoral and/or unethical fantasies. Our focus is on healthy dreams that can improve our physical, mental, emotional and spiritual health.

If you're still having trouble believing that a major lifestyle change might be just the medicine you need to heal your life, I encourage you to read Dr. LeShan's book (any bookstore can order it for you if they don't have it in stock; I ordered my copy from amazon.com). Trust me, you'll be a believer.

Whatever your dream is – small or spectacular – you can achieve it if you will only believe that you can and take the first steps toward it. After those first few scary steps, momentum will carry you forward. Hey, you've survived cancer! Everything is possible now, isn't it?

We never took vacations before cancer entered our lives. Now, in addition to our trips to the beach, we take *adventures* whenever we can. We took a cruise up the Mississippi River on the paddlewheel steamboat "Delta Queen" and another one across the Gulf of Mexico, skirting a hurricane all the way, ending up in a small coastal town in Mexico (the hurricane kept us from our destination of Cancun) where the residents were so excited to see a cruise ship that the whole town turned out and threw a party on the dock, complete with a band and dancers. We've gone parasailing and jet skiing. Roger flew an airplane, and I rode a Harley-Davidson. We've traveled to exciting places like Las Vegas and beautiful spots like the Berkshires and Bermuda. We went swimming with dolphins in Florida. And of course we ran the Marine Corps Marathon. Future plans include a wilderness adventure and another marathon, and a cross-country road trip traveling as far as we can go on the legendary Route 66.

These may not seem like adventures to a lot of people, but they are for us. It doesn't have to be full of heart-stopping action to be an adventure. What matters is that you do the things *you* want to do.

Some readers who are currently in treatment undoubtedly are saying or thinking at this point *Well, this certainly isn't for me. I am far too ill to be thinking about living my dreams or taking a road trip or redecorating my house.*

We are not so naïve or such pie-in-the-sky dreamers or so far out from our own cancer experiences that we don't understand these huge lifestyle changes may be far more than some cancer patients can manage *right now*. But that doesn't mean those same patients won't be able to manage these or other changes later on. We couldn't have trained for or run a marathon during our treatments or even a year or two later. We ran the Marine Corps Marathon four years after we were diagnosed with and treated for our cancers.

Whatever the current state of your health, *focus on the future*. If you're confined to bed or home right now, write out your plans for what you're going to do when you're well. If you're not well enough to write, talk about your plans with a family member or friend and ask them to take notes for you.

Family reunion? Write out the menu. Going on a cruise? Plan your wardrobe. Thinking about a new career or hobby? List the items you'll need to buy and study. Read everything you can about the subjects or places you plan to explore when you're on your feet again. Use this time to plan and prepare for the major lifestyle changes you want to make when you're well.

By the way, we know of one gentleman who was hospitalized on a number of occasions and considered "critical" more than once during his two-year battle with cancer. He had worked for the railroad for forty-nine of his sixty-four years, but he had harbored a secret fantasy of learning to play the banjo. On one of his good days, he decided if that dream was ever going to come true, he had better get started on it. So his wife found a local banjo player who was willing to come to the house and even to the hospital to give him lessons. The last we heard, he was picking and singing his heart out at county fairs and other events up and down the east coast, performing while square dancers and cloggers dance, and sometimes entertaining audiences by himself, singing original songs while accompanying himself on the banjo.

The "something amazing" you choose will determine what your legacy will be. No matter how long your life, the generations that come after you will know you for the man, woman or child who "_____ _____ (fill in the blank with your own amazing accomplishment) when she had cancer" or "after he recovered from cancer."

When you consider your legacy, remember the priceless gift of understanding you have received, the gift of living, laughing and loving fully through every moment of every day remaining to you because you have accepted and are at peace with the fact that we are all mortal. You have learned so much on this journey, and the way in which you share the knowledge and deep understanding you have gained at such a dear price becomes part of your legacy, too.

Of all the many things you've learned, perhaps the most important is that courage doesn't mean the absence of fear. It means feeling the fear, and running headlong into the fight anyway.

Remember what Eleanor Roosevelt said: "You gain strength, courage and confidence every time you stop to look fear in the face...You must do the thing you think you cannot do."

You *can* do it. You *must* do it.

You are a soldier in the war on cancer. Fight on, brave warrior.

Please visit The Cancer Crusade's website at
www.TheCancerCrusade.com and sign up for
the free monthly online newsletter, "The Cancer
Connection."

And please take a few minutes to view the powerful
"Survivor Movie" at www.TheSurvivorMovie.com.
As this book goes to print, this little movie has been
viewed nearly 200,000 times in more than 30 coun-
tries. It is changing the lives of cancer survivors and
caregivers around the world. More than 3,000 of
them have written just to say "Thank you!"

We hope you will write to us to share your personal stories as well as your thoughts about our
publications and "The Survivor Movie."

To order additional copies of *Medicine, Marathons
and Miracles: Turning a Diagnosis of Cancer into
Personal Victory*, please contact:

Roger and Kathy Cawthon
The Cancer Crusade
1 Felton Place
Hampton, VA 23666
757.826.7513
www.TheCancerCrusade.com
cawthons@TheCancerCrusade.com